Sexy Anime Girls

Coloring Book for Grown-Ups 1

UNCENSORED

ColoringArtist.com

Adults Coloring Books

Angel Flower Girl Coloring Book 1

Anime Coloring Book 1

Aztec Coloring Book 1

Cartoons Coloring Book for Grown-Ups 1

Churches Coloring Book for Grown-Ups 1

Dazzling Doodles Coloring Book for Grown-Ups 1

Desserts and Cupcakes Coloring Book for Grown-Ups 1

Dreamcatchers Coloring Book for Grown-Ups 1

Dreamy Doodles Coloring Book for Grown-Ups 1

Enchanted Coloring Book for Grown-Ups 1

Funky People Coloring Book for Grown-Ups 1

Guns Coloring Book for Grown-Ups 1

Hot Air Balloons Coloring Book for Grown-Ups 1

Houses Coloring Book for Grown-Ups 1

Lighthouses Coloring Book for Grown-Ups 1

Mermaids Coloring Book for Grown-Ups 1

Monsters Coloring Book for Grown-Ups 1

Mushrooms Coloring Book for Grown-Ups 1

Occult Coloring Book for Grown-Ups 1

Pop Art Coloring Book for Grown-Ups 1

Robots Coloring Book for Grown-Ups 1

Russian Dolls Coloring Book for Grown-Ups 1

Sexy Girls Coloring Book for Grown-Ups 1

Sexy Waitress Coloring Book 1

Skulls Coloring Book for Grown-Ups 1

Smileys Coloring Book for Grown-Ups 1

Steampunk Coloring Book 1

Steampunk Girls Coloring Book for Grown-Ups 1

Tarot Cards Coloring Book for Grown-Ups 1

Wild West Cowboys and Cowgirls Coloring Book for Grown-Ups 1

Wonderful World Coloring Book for Grown-Ups 1

Yoga Coloring Book for Grown-Ups 1

Zodiac Signs Coloring Book for Grown-Ups 1

Zombie Coloring Book 1

Copyright © 2016 - Nick Snels
Cover by Slamet Hariyadi
http://www.coloringartist.com

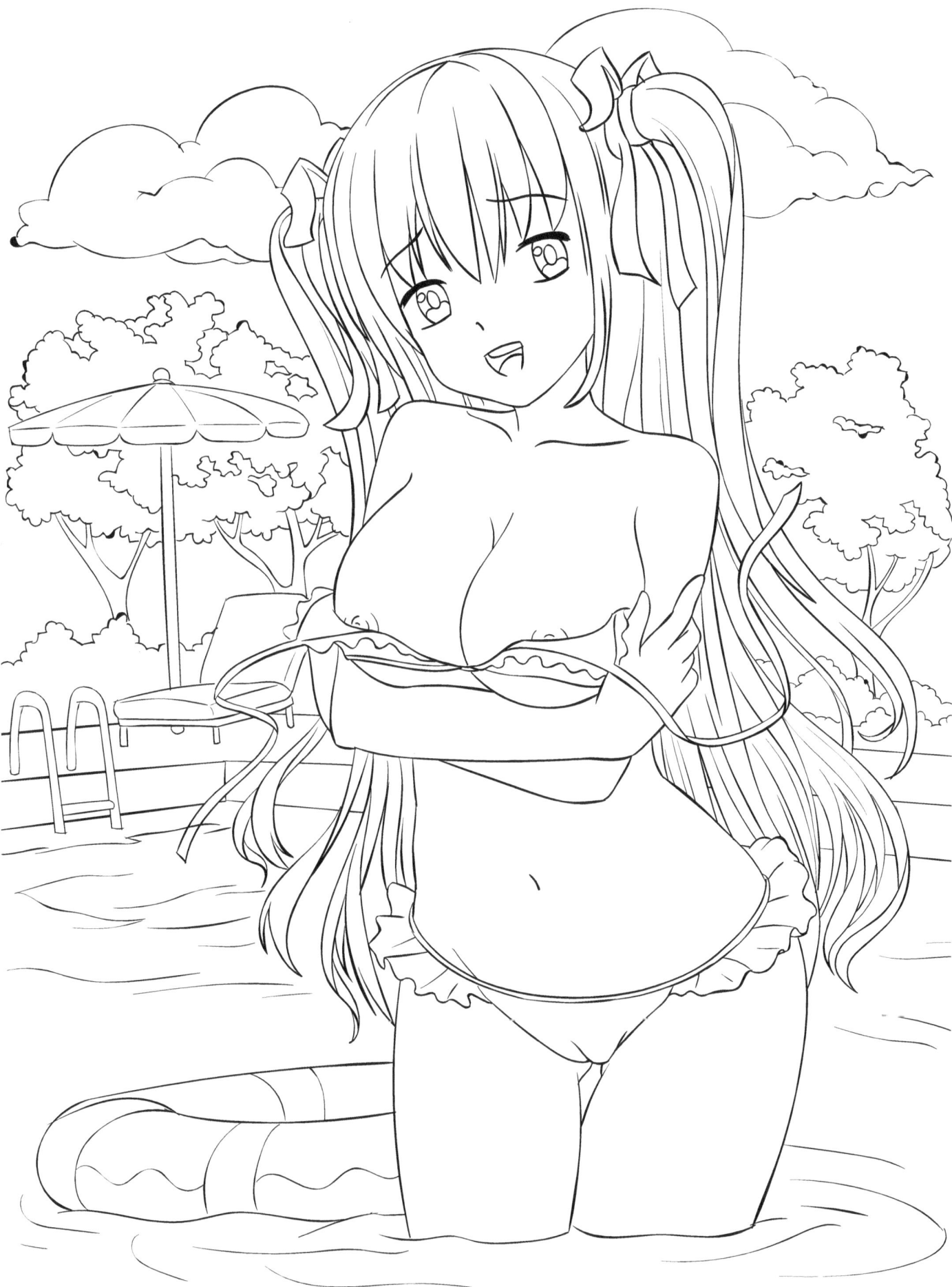

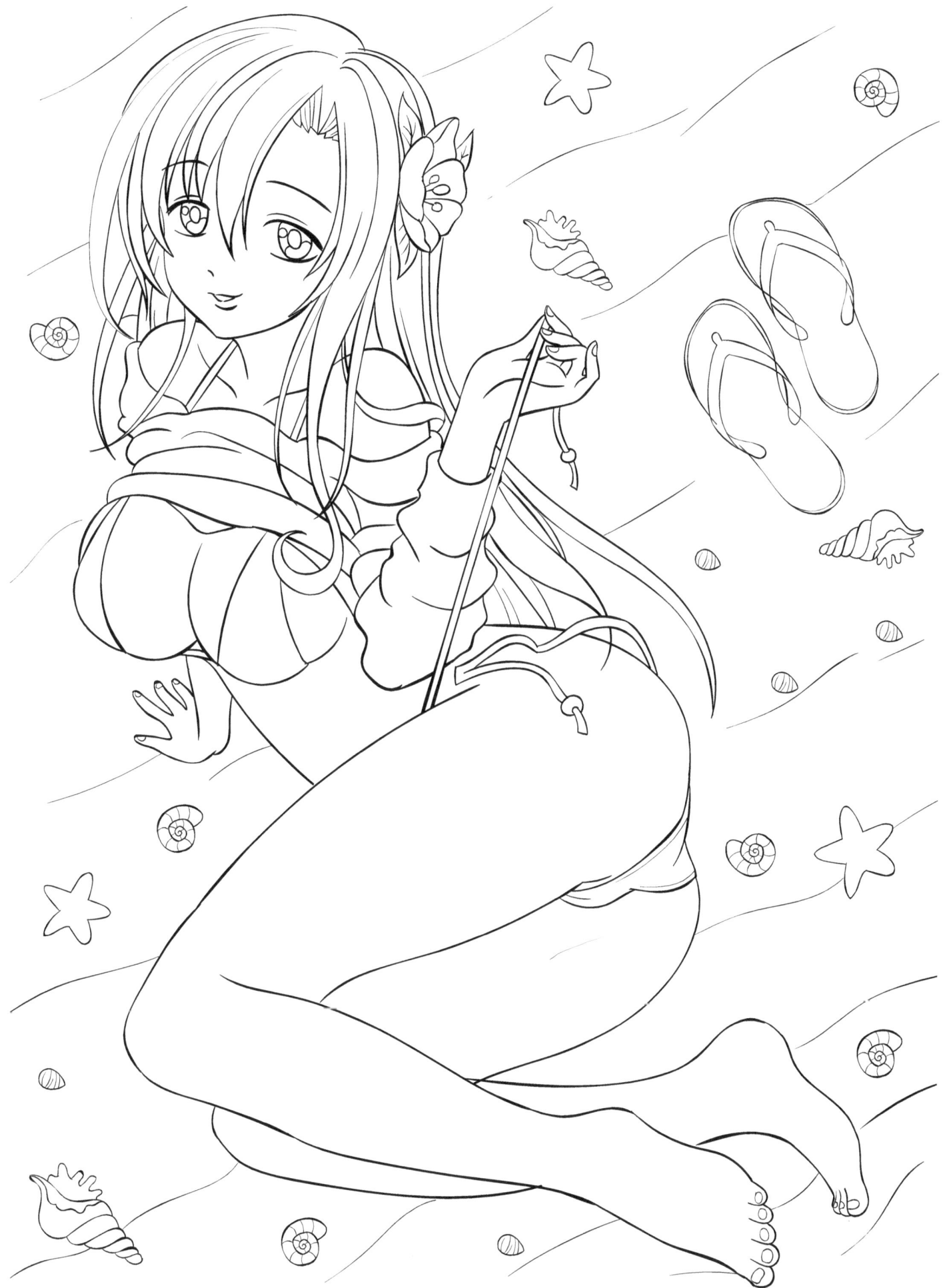

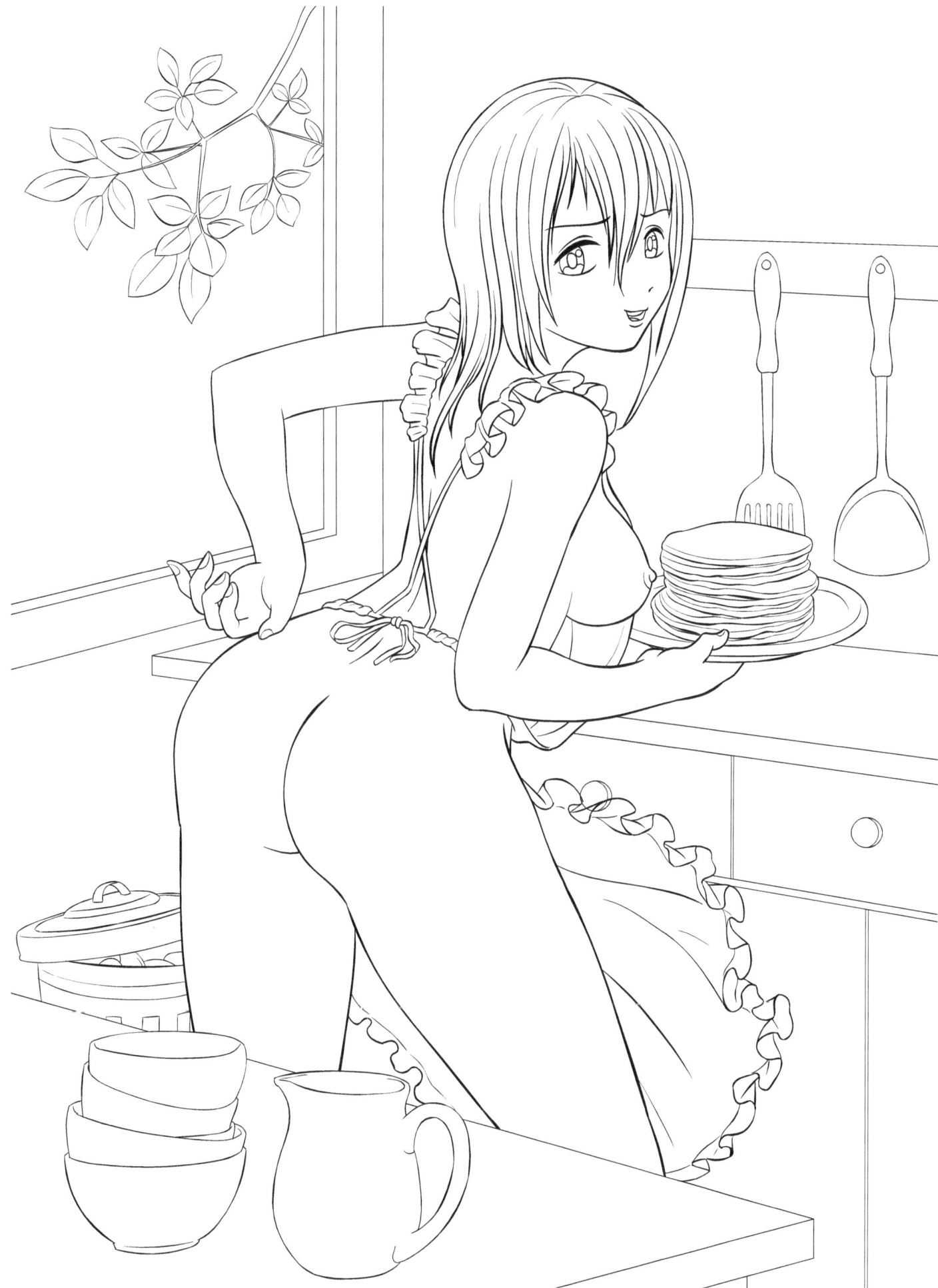

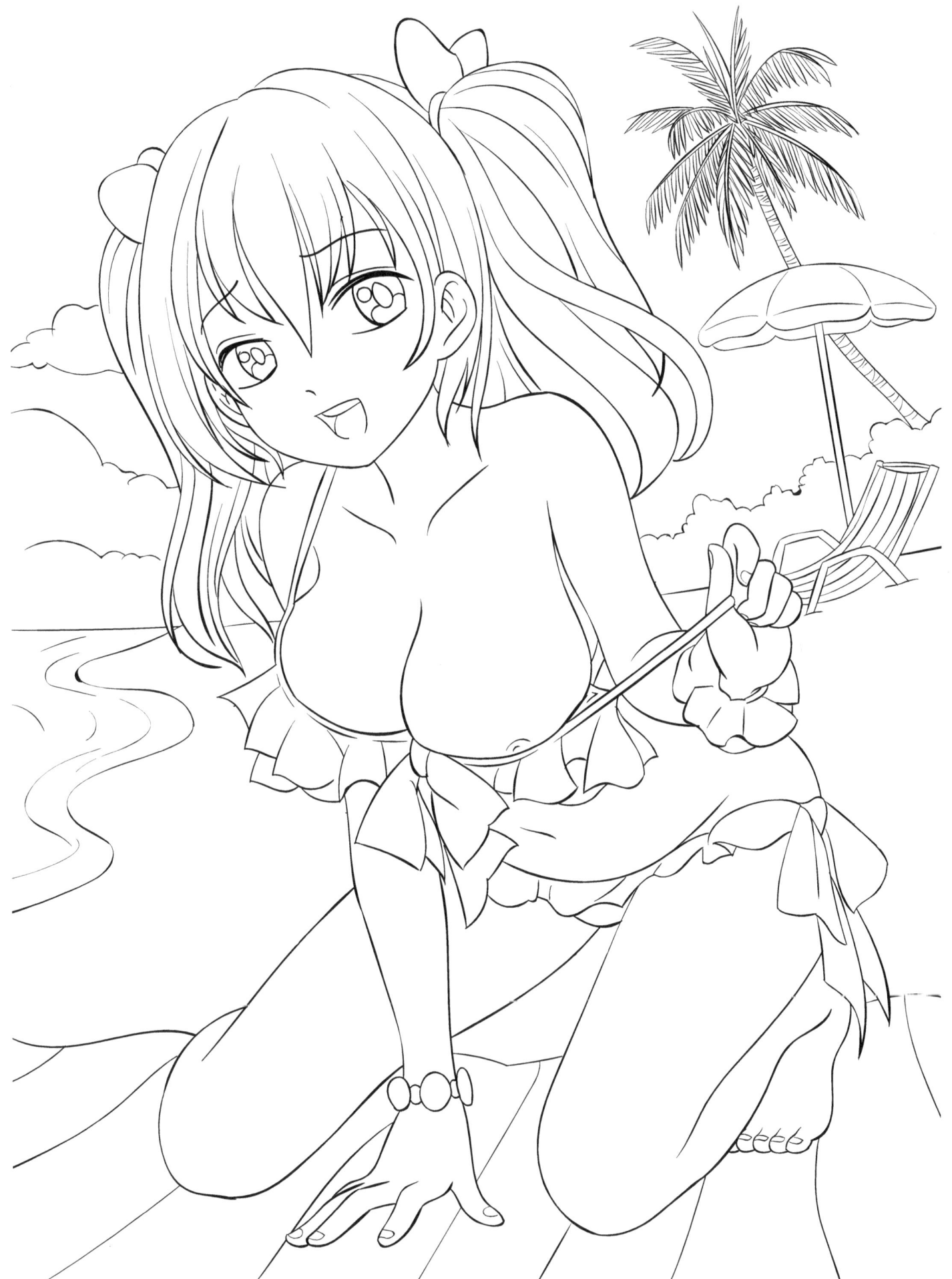

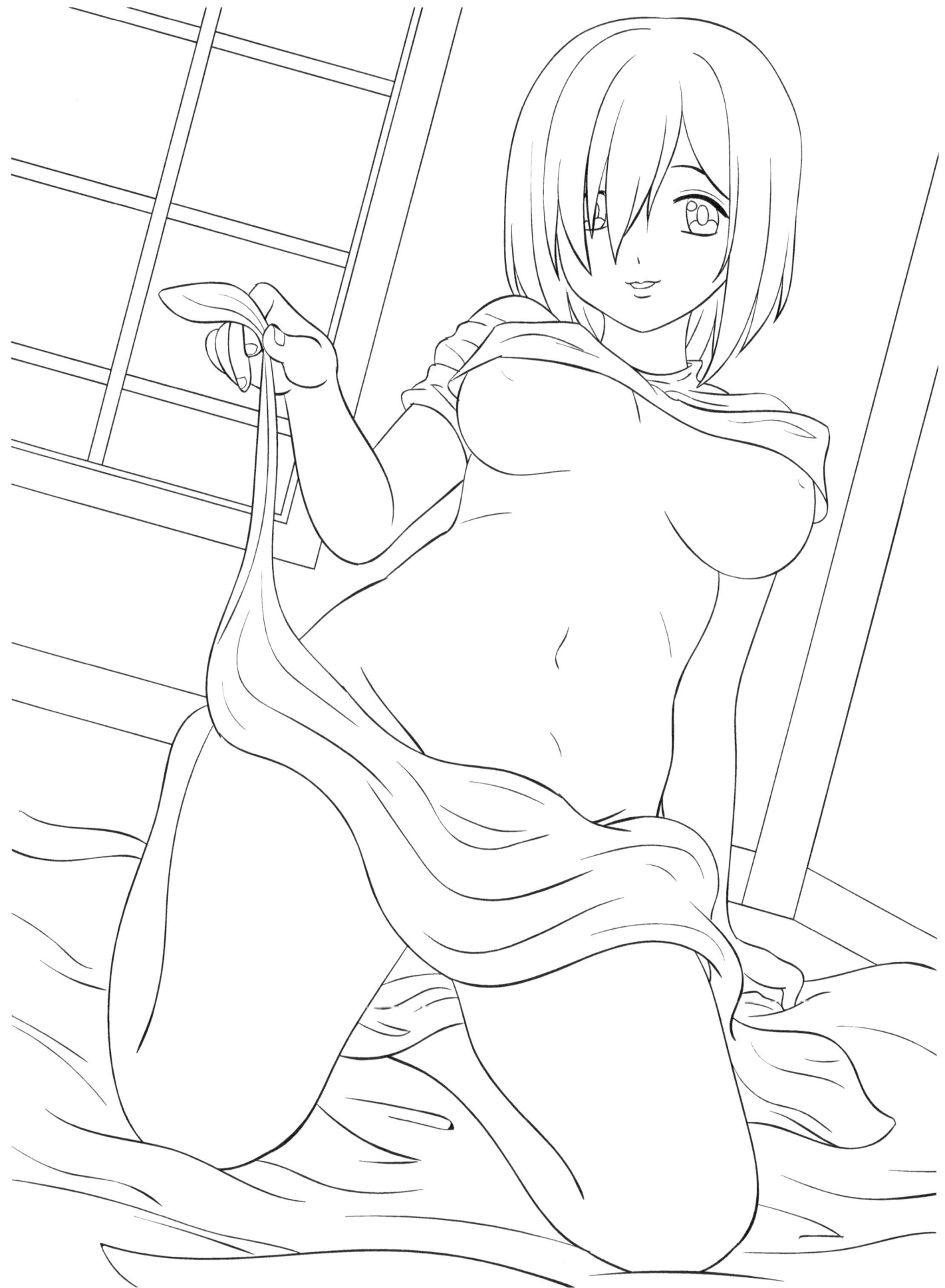

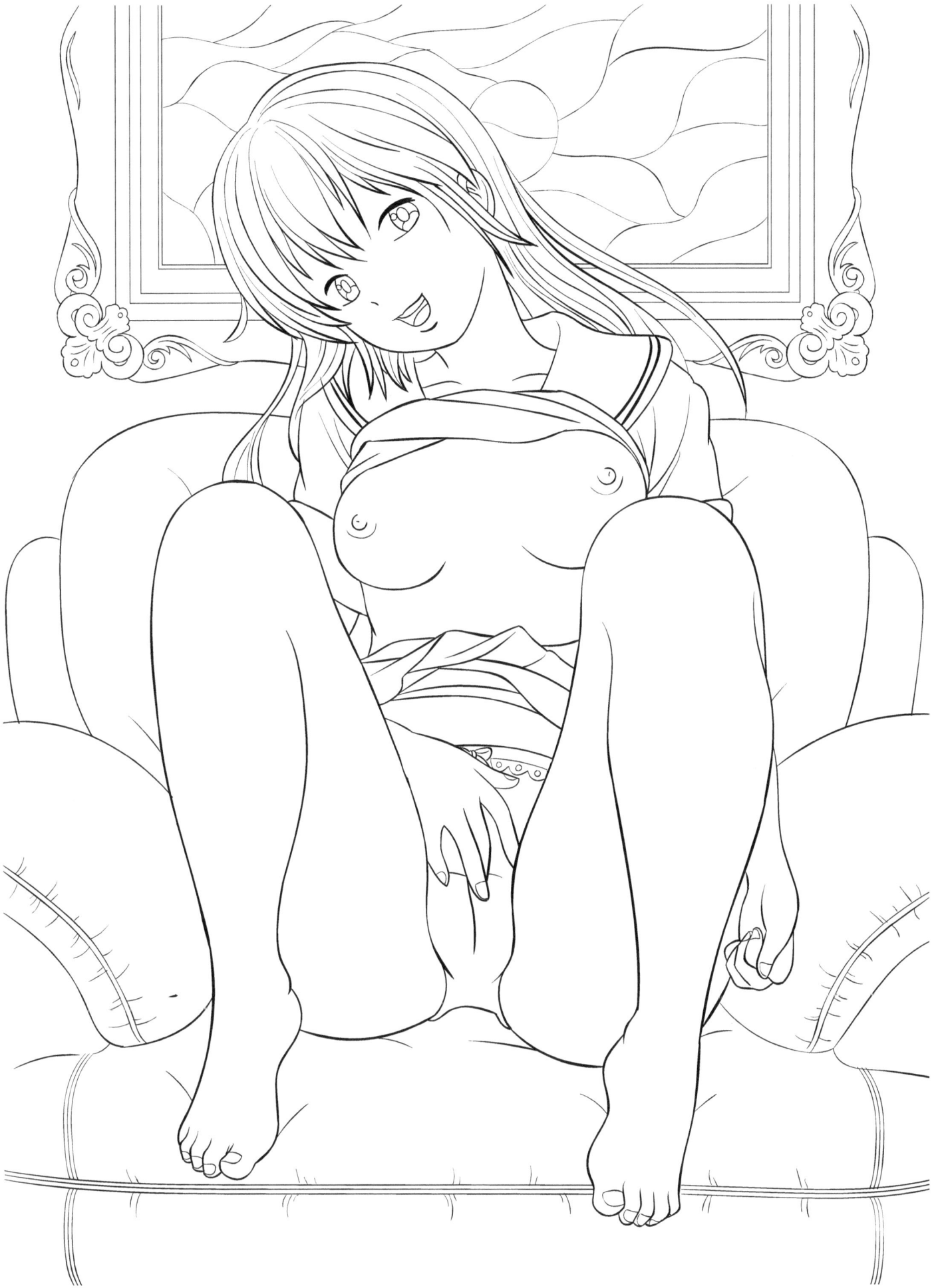

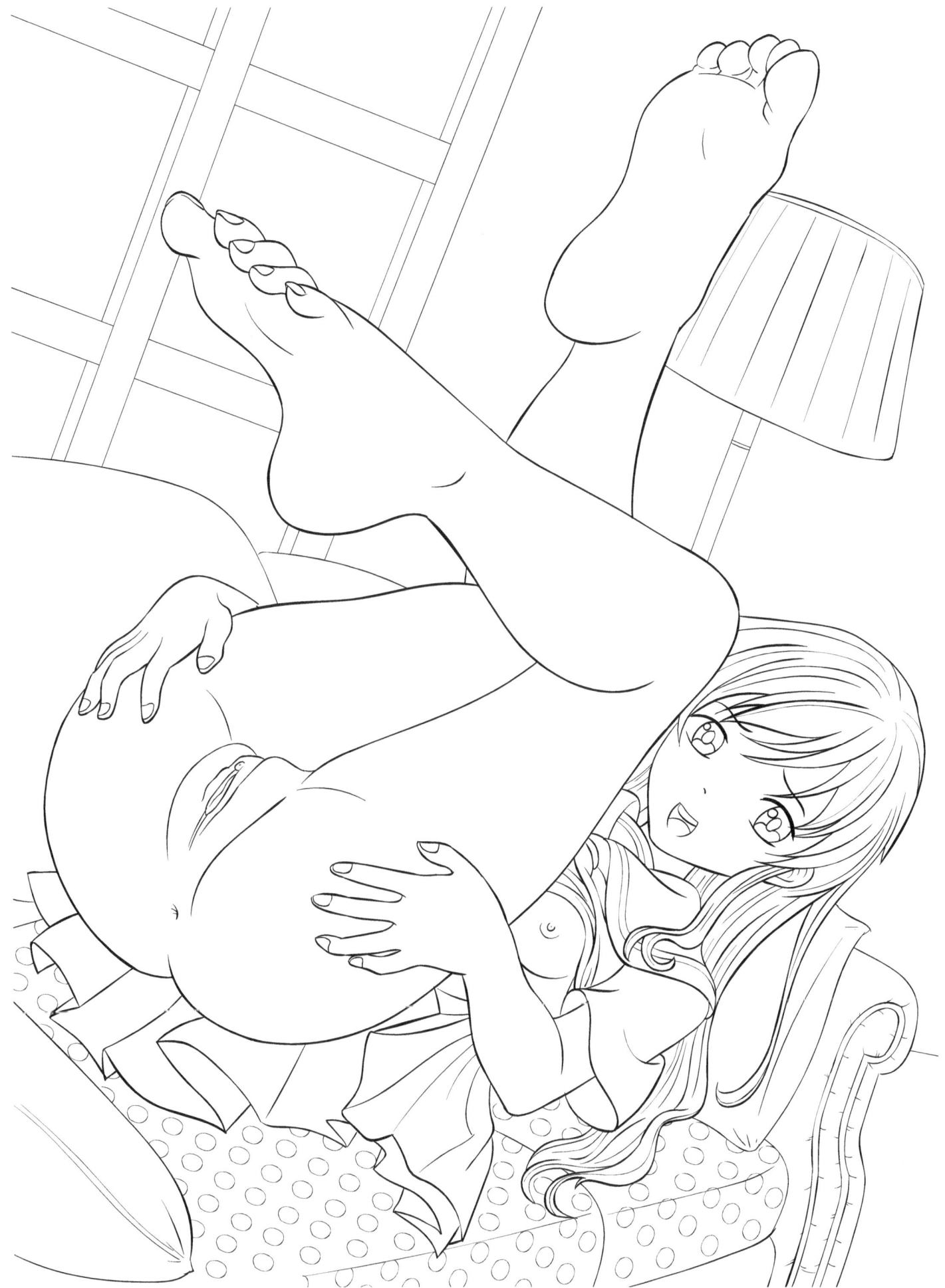

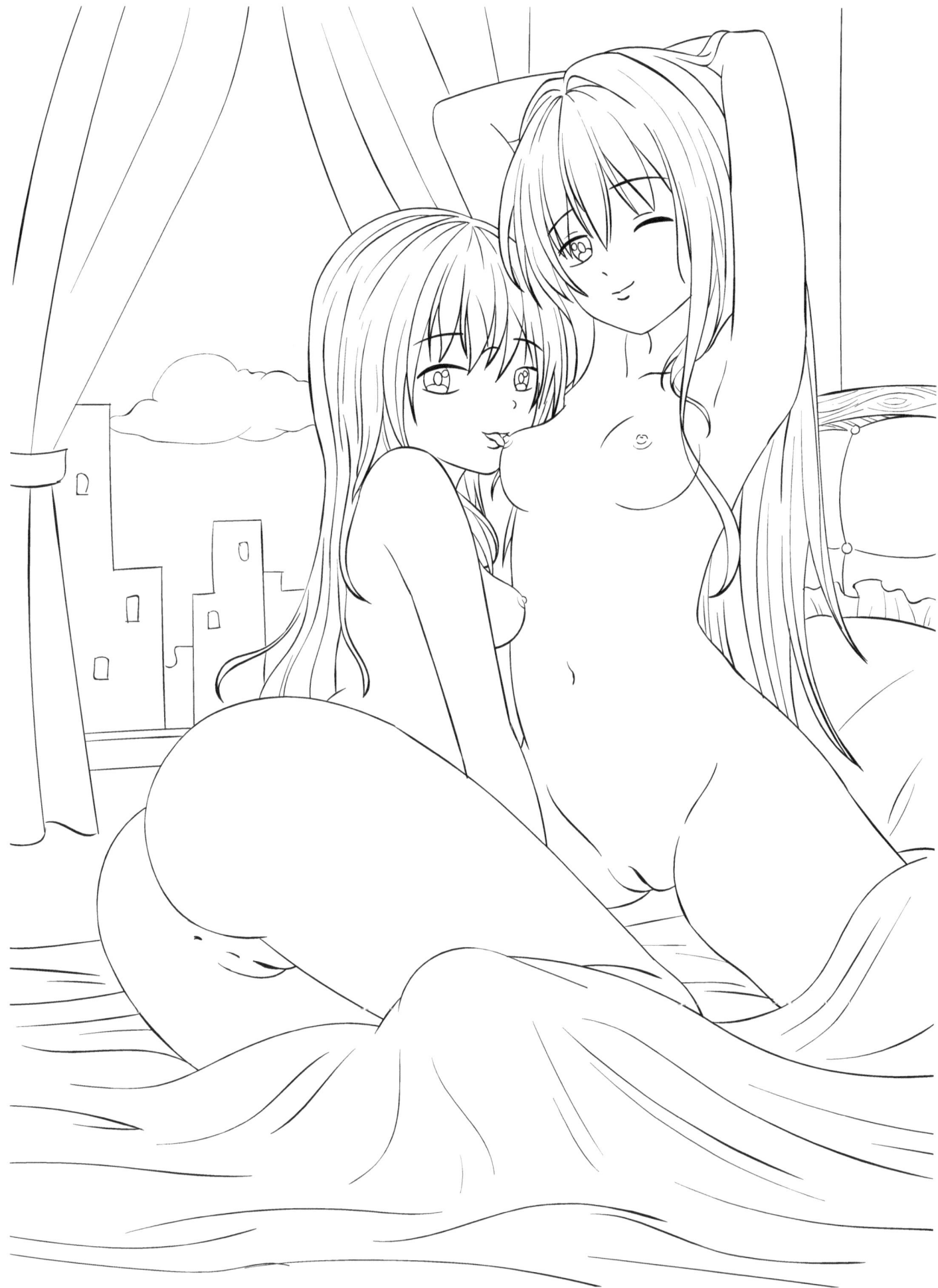

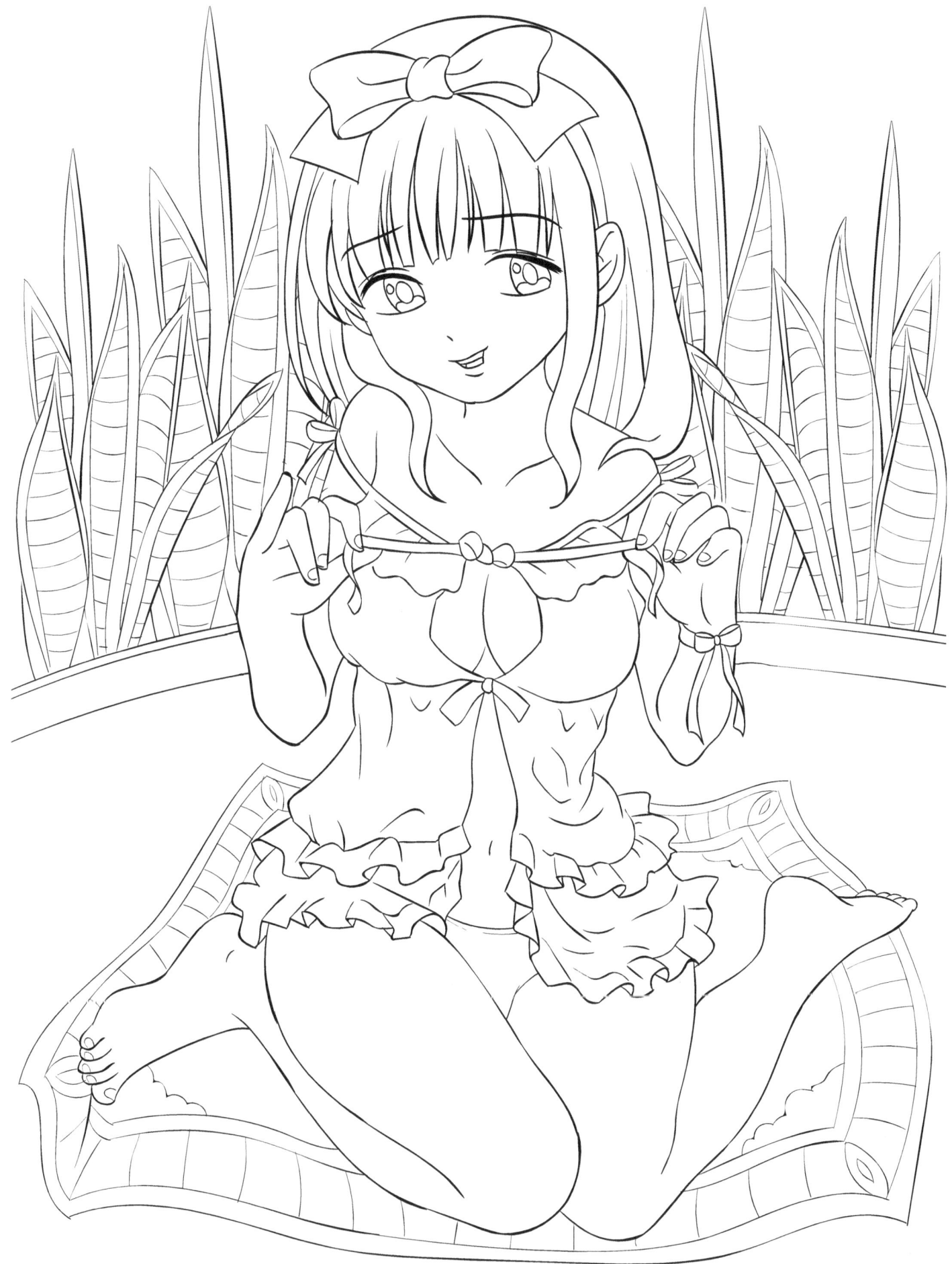

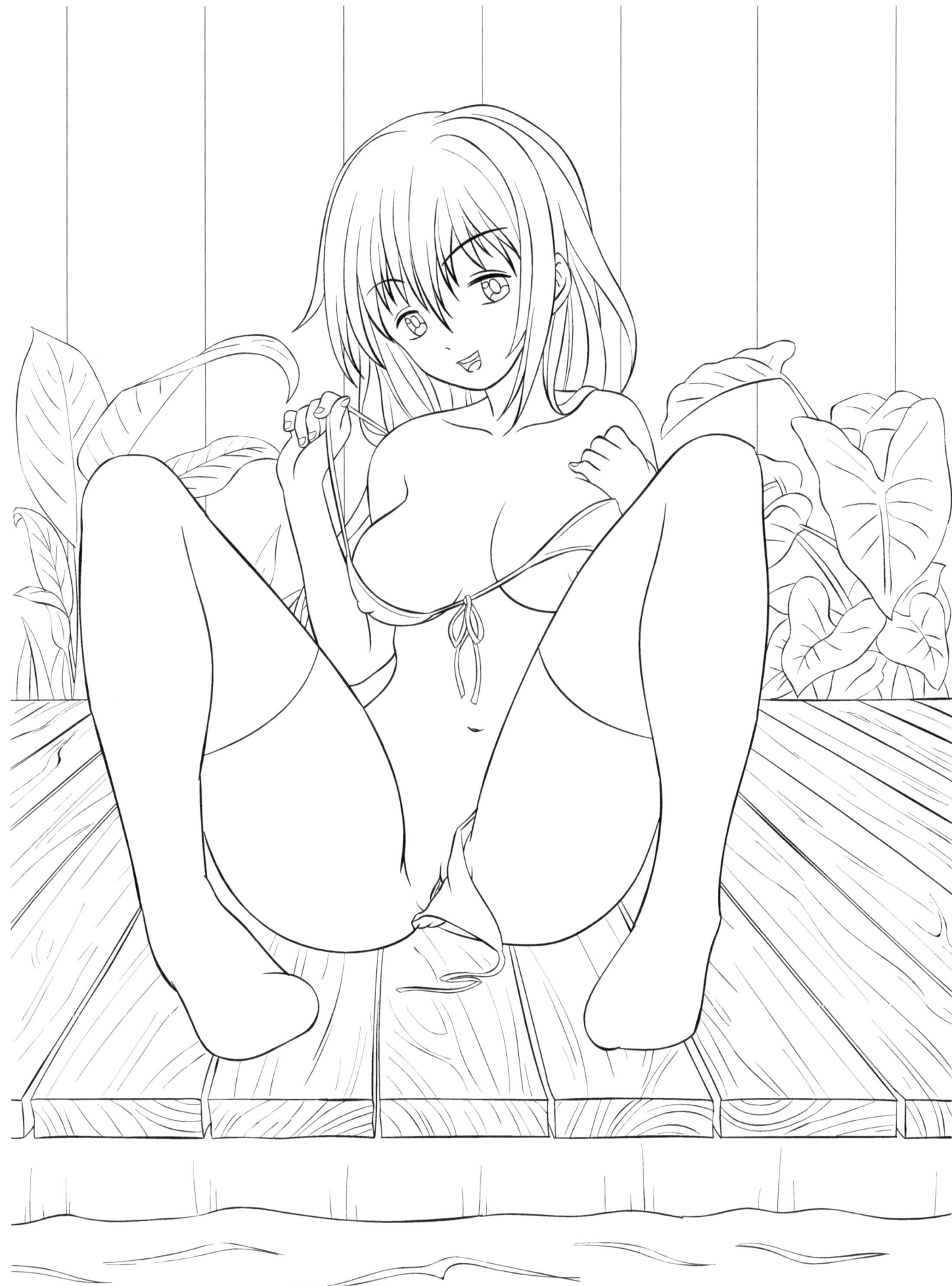

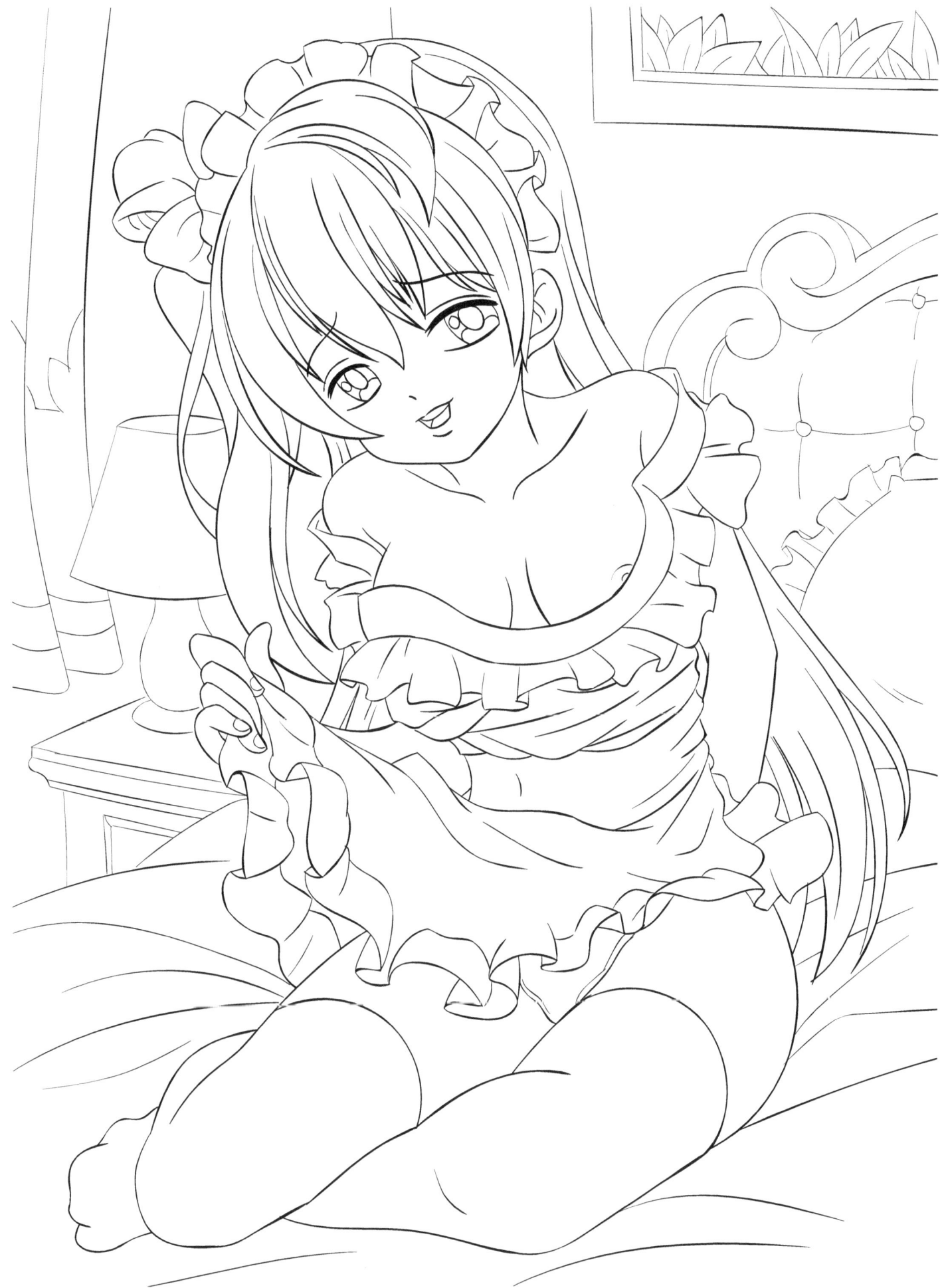

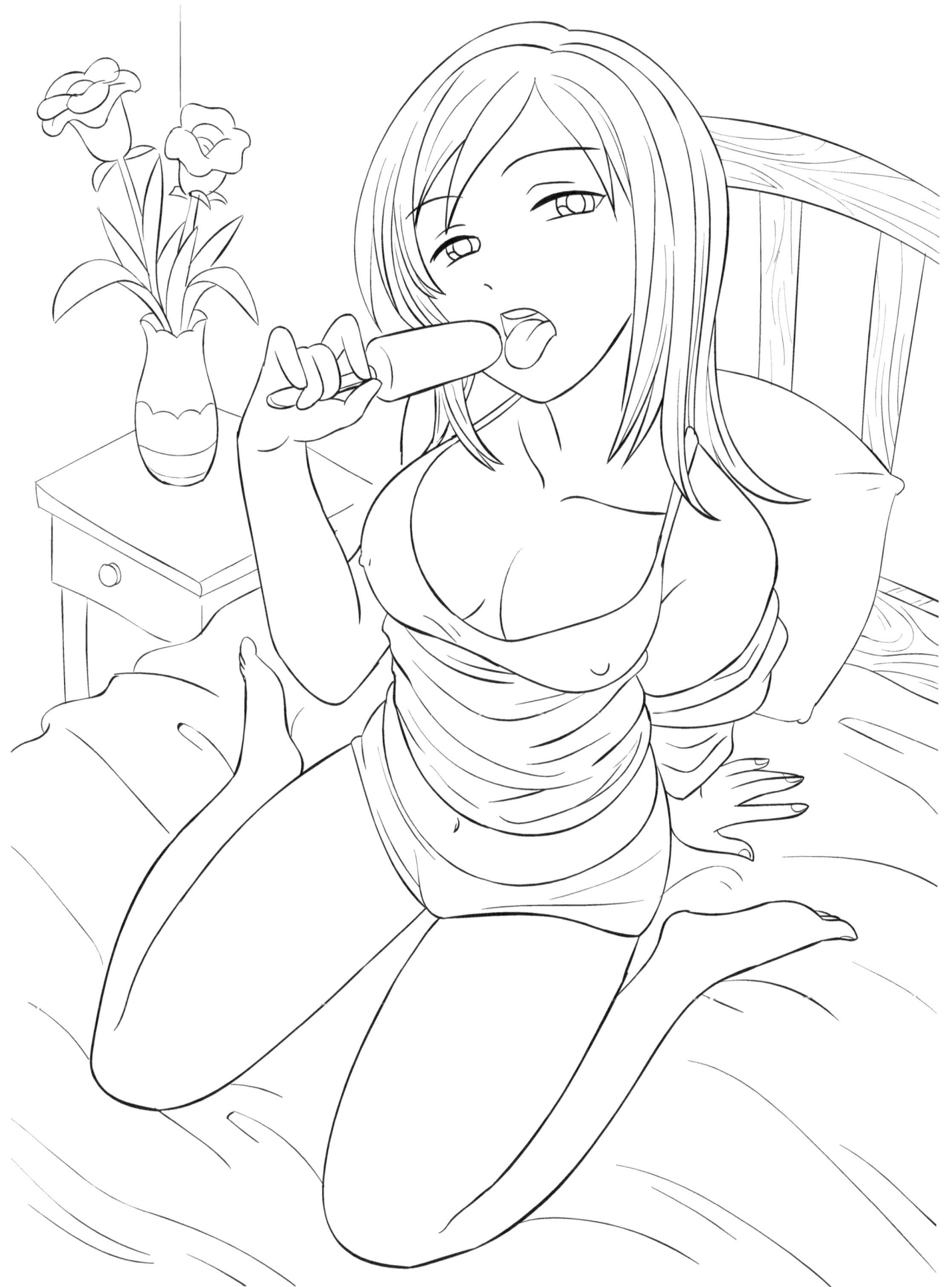

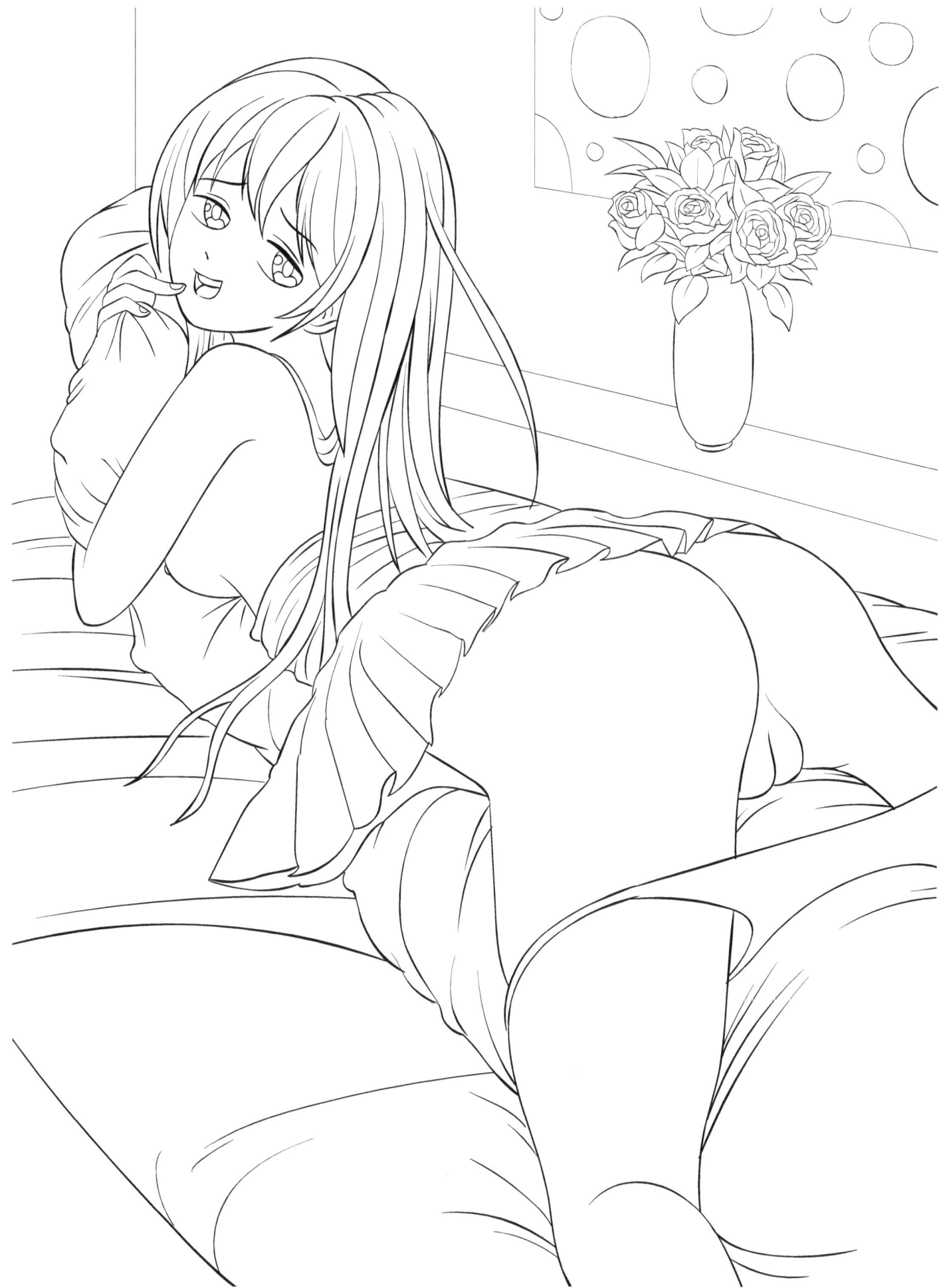

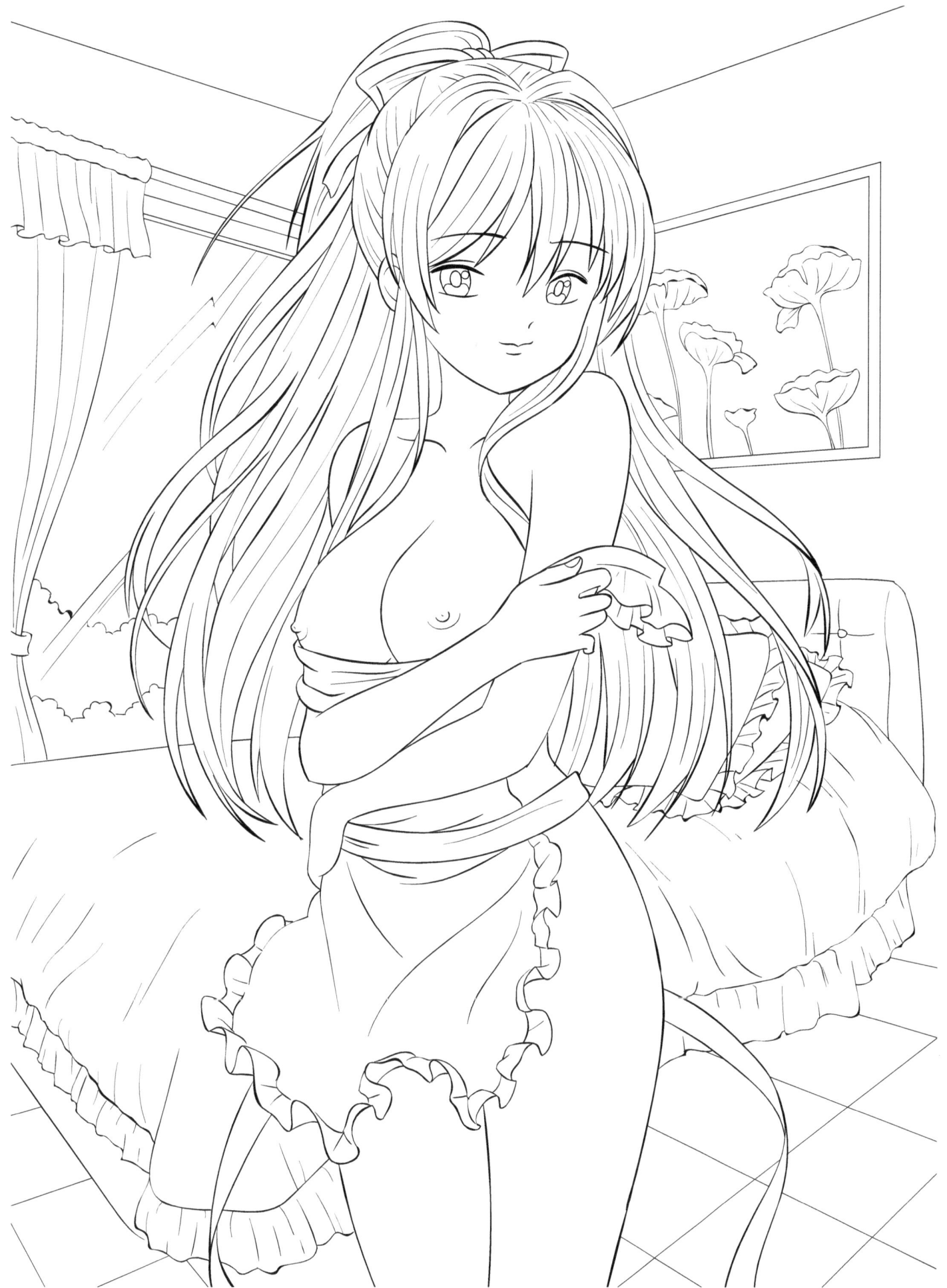

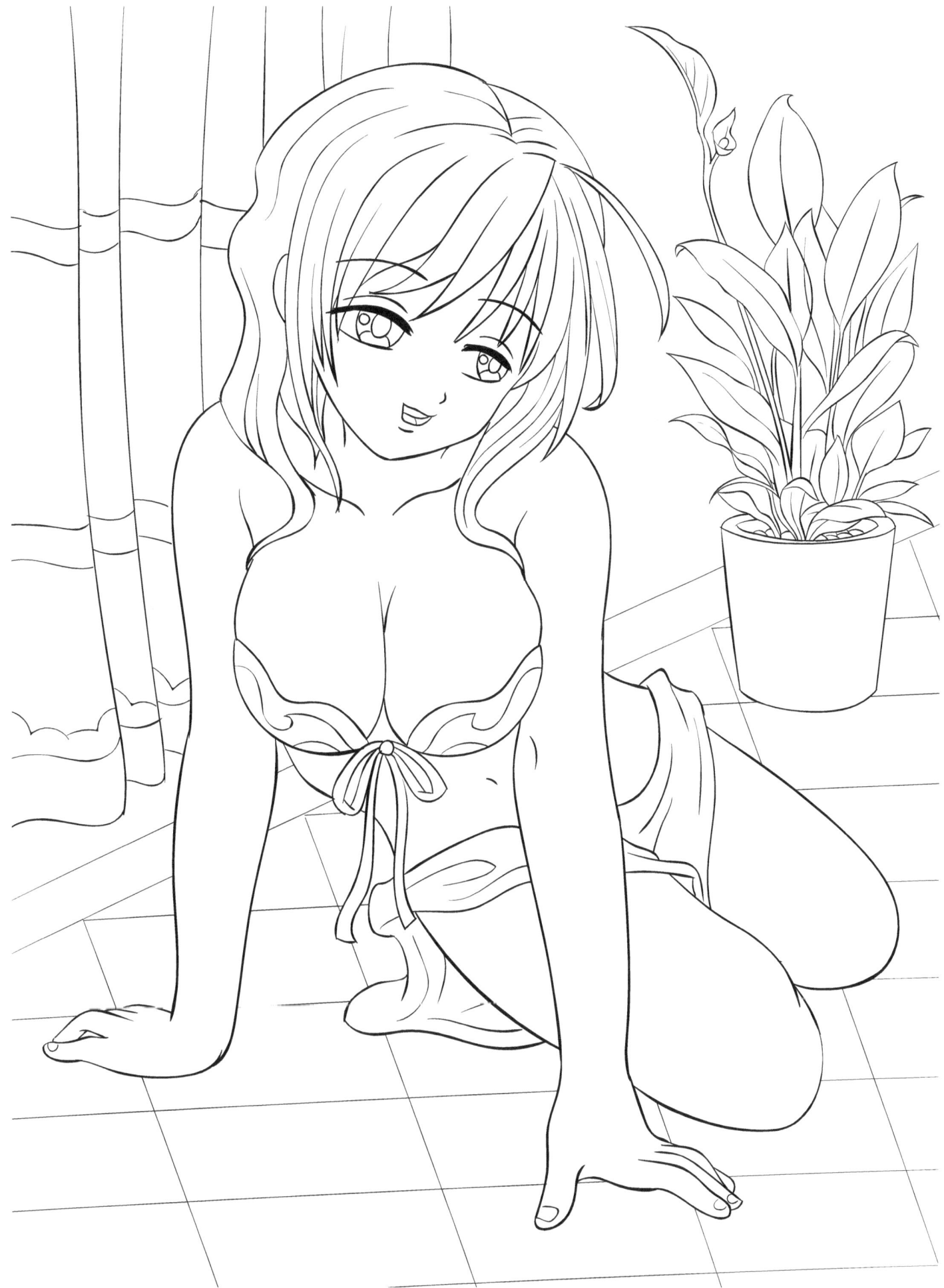

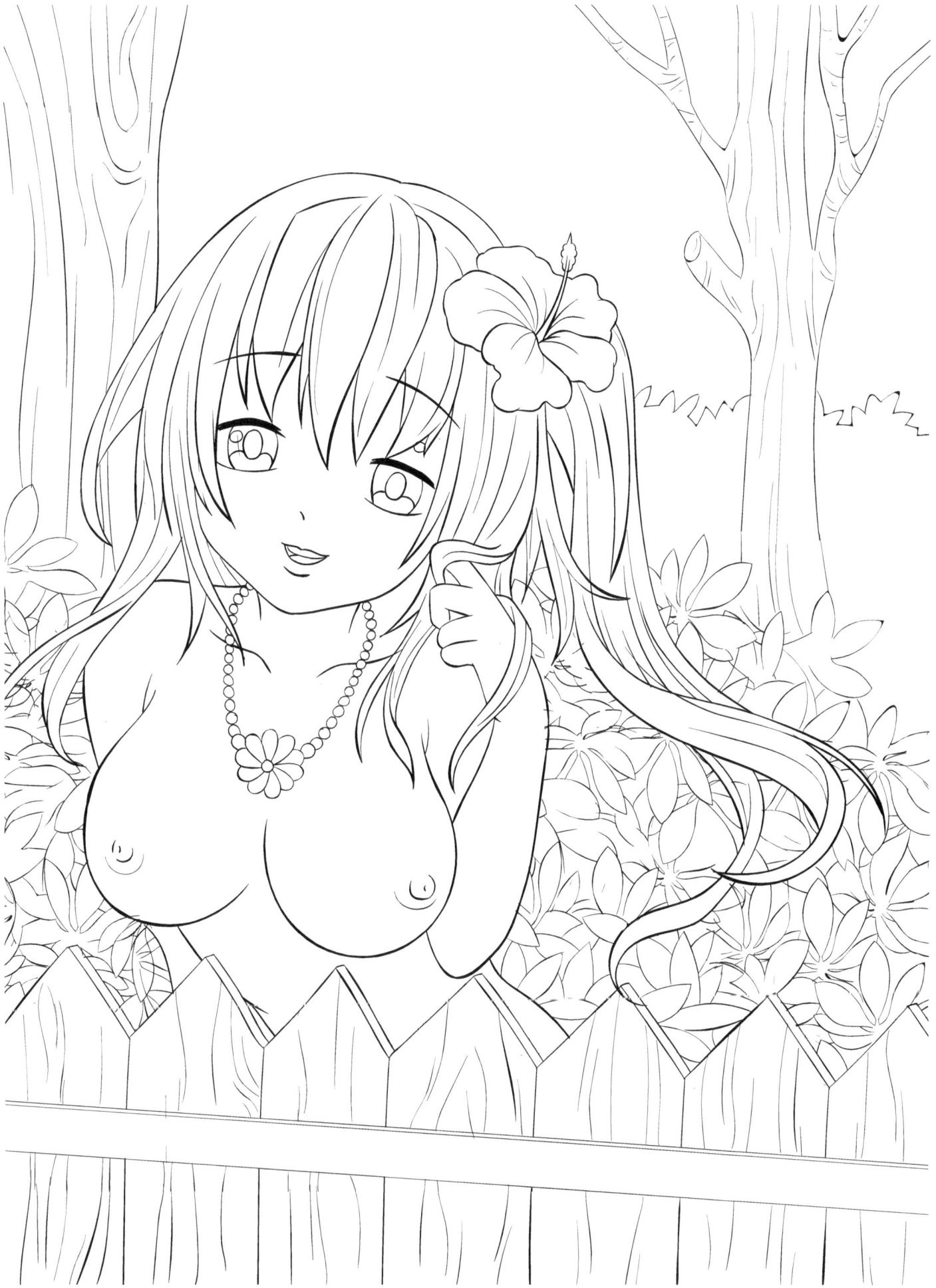

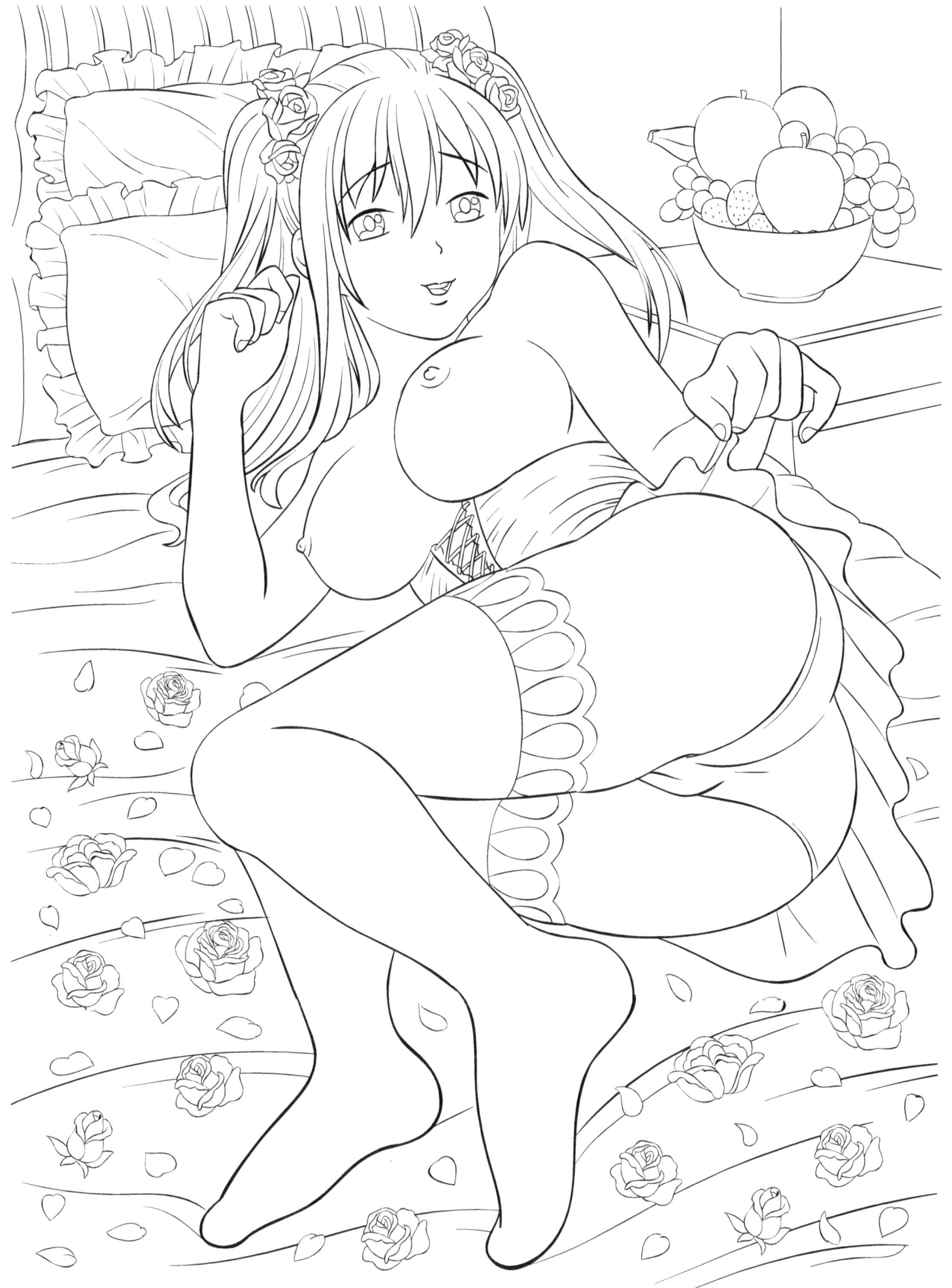

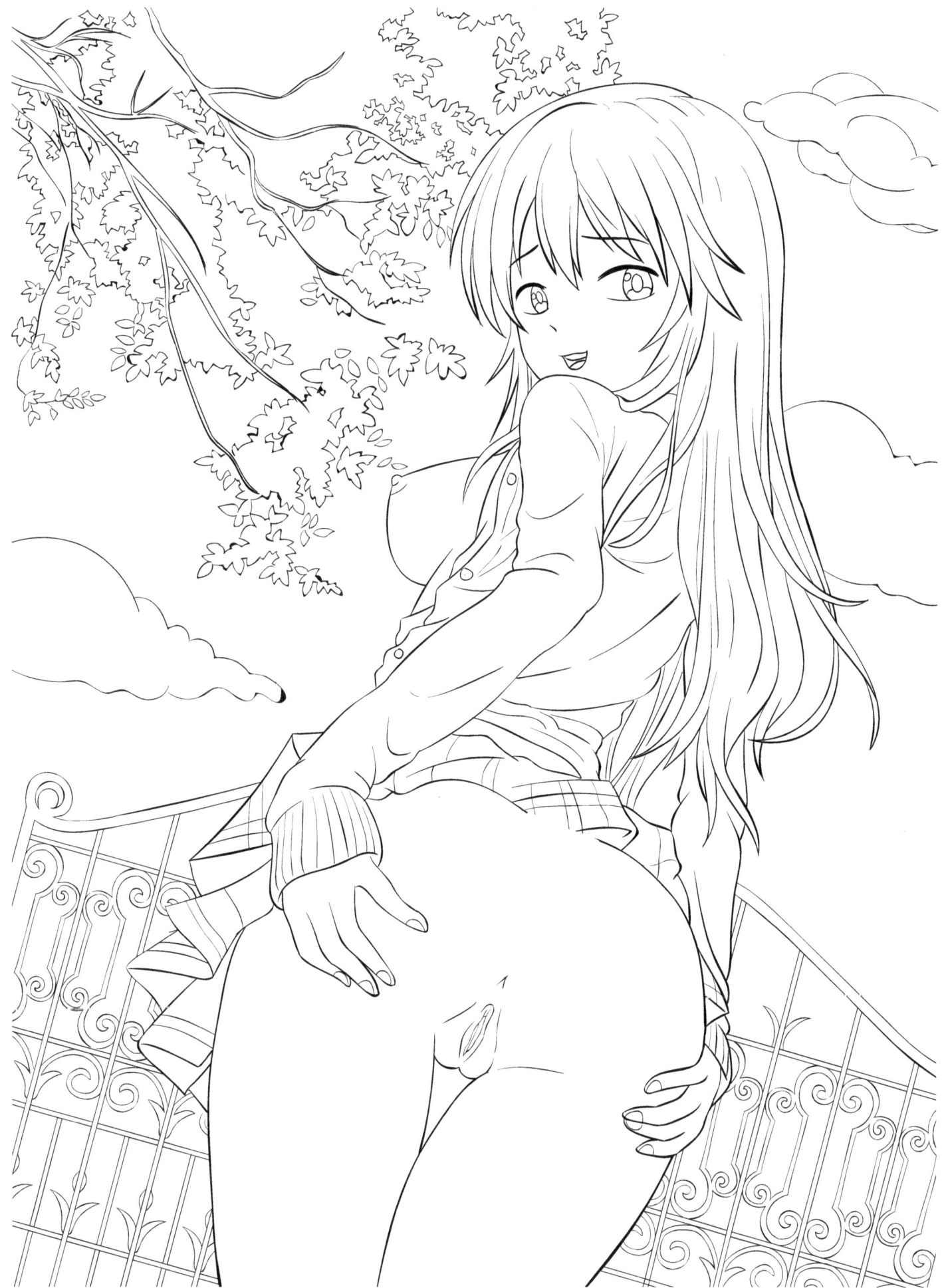

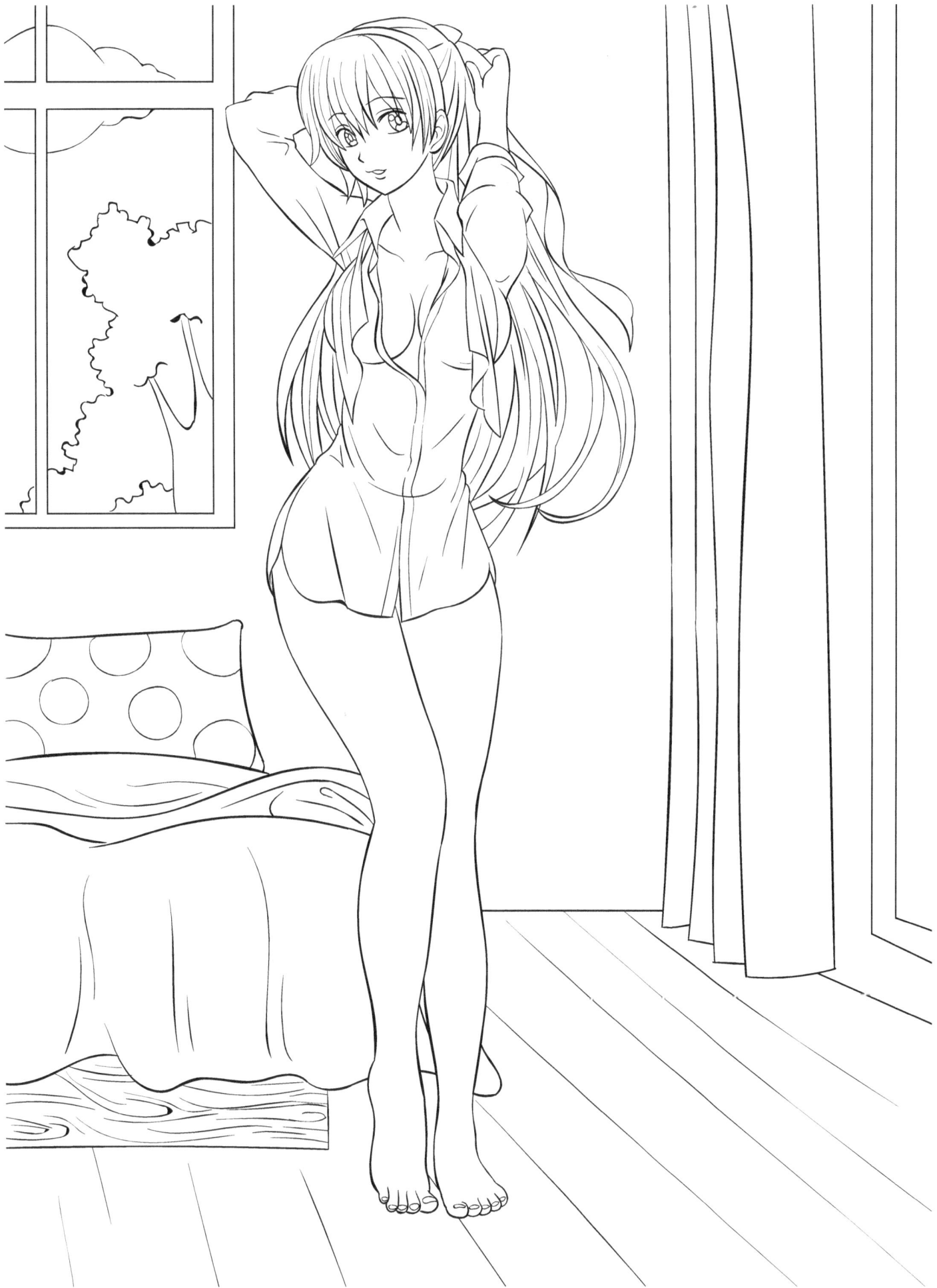

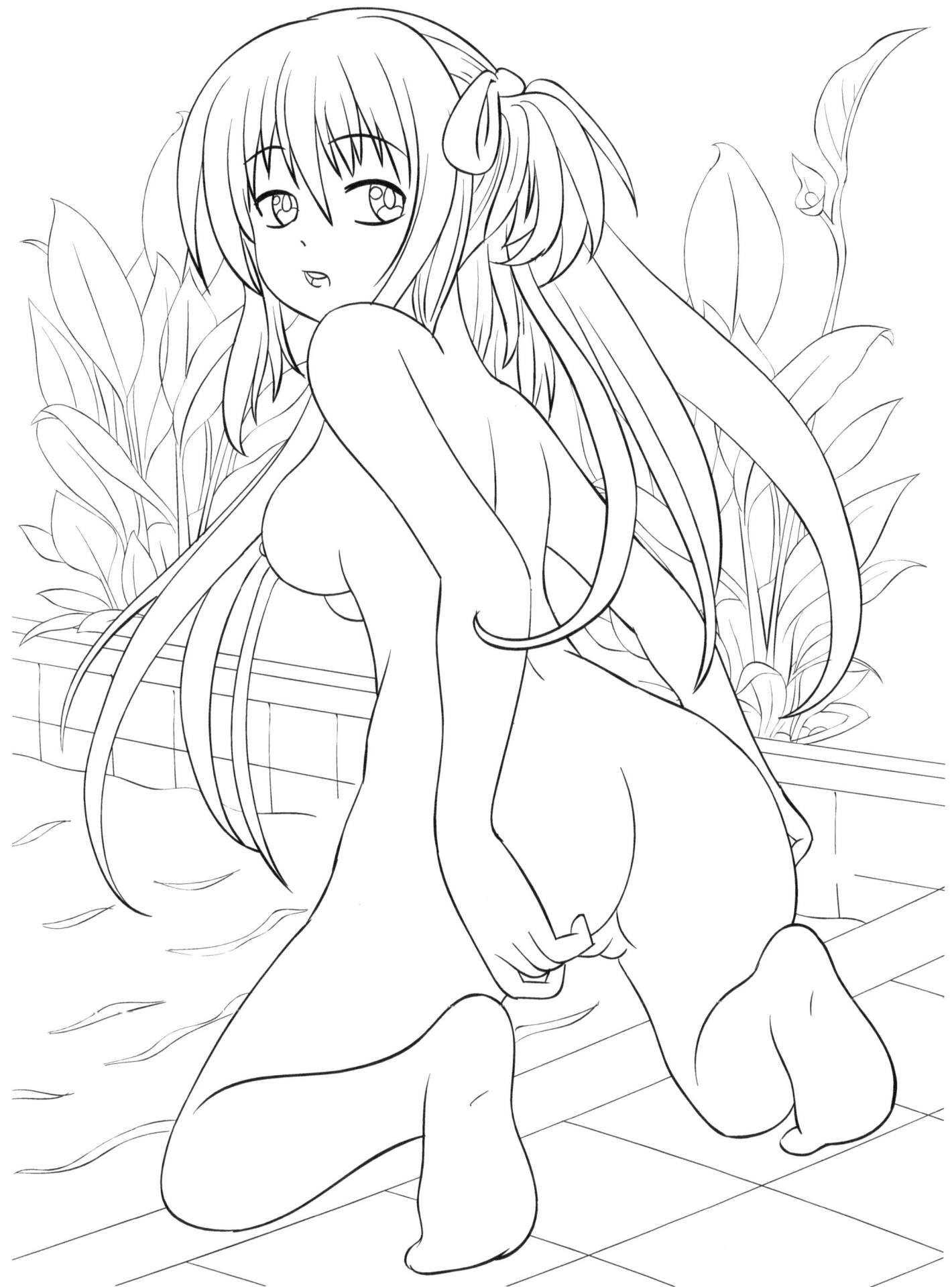

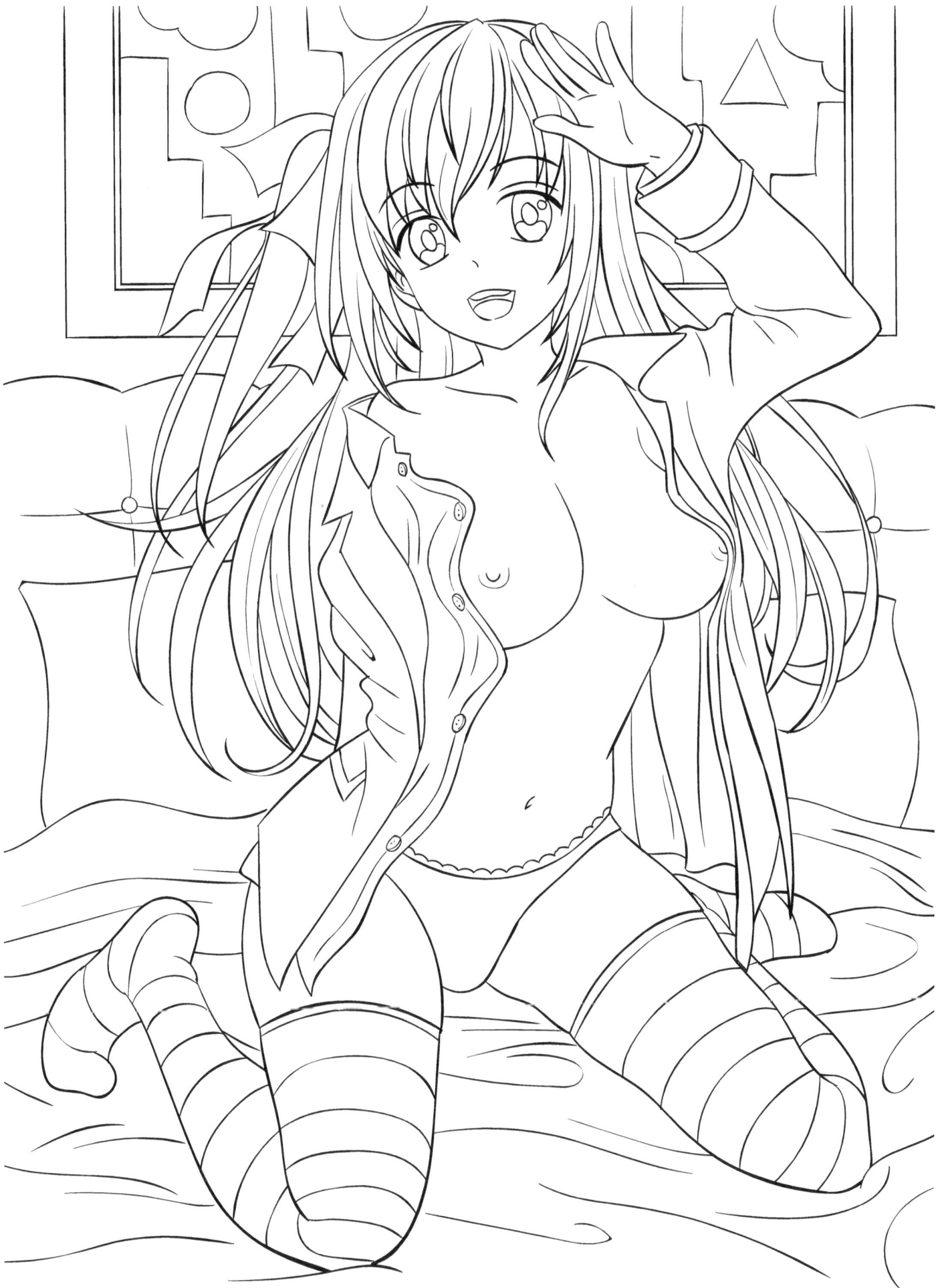

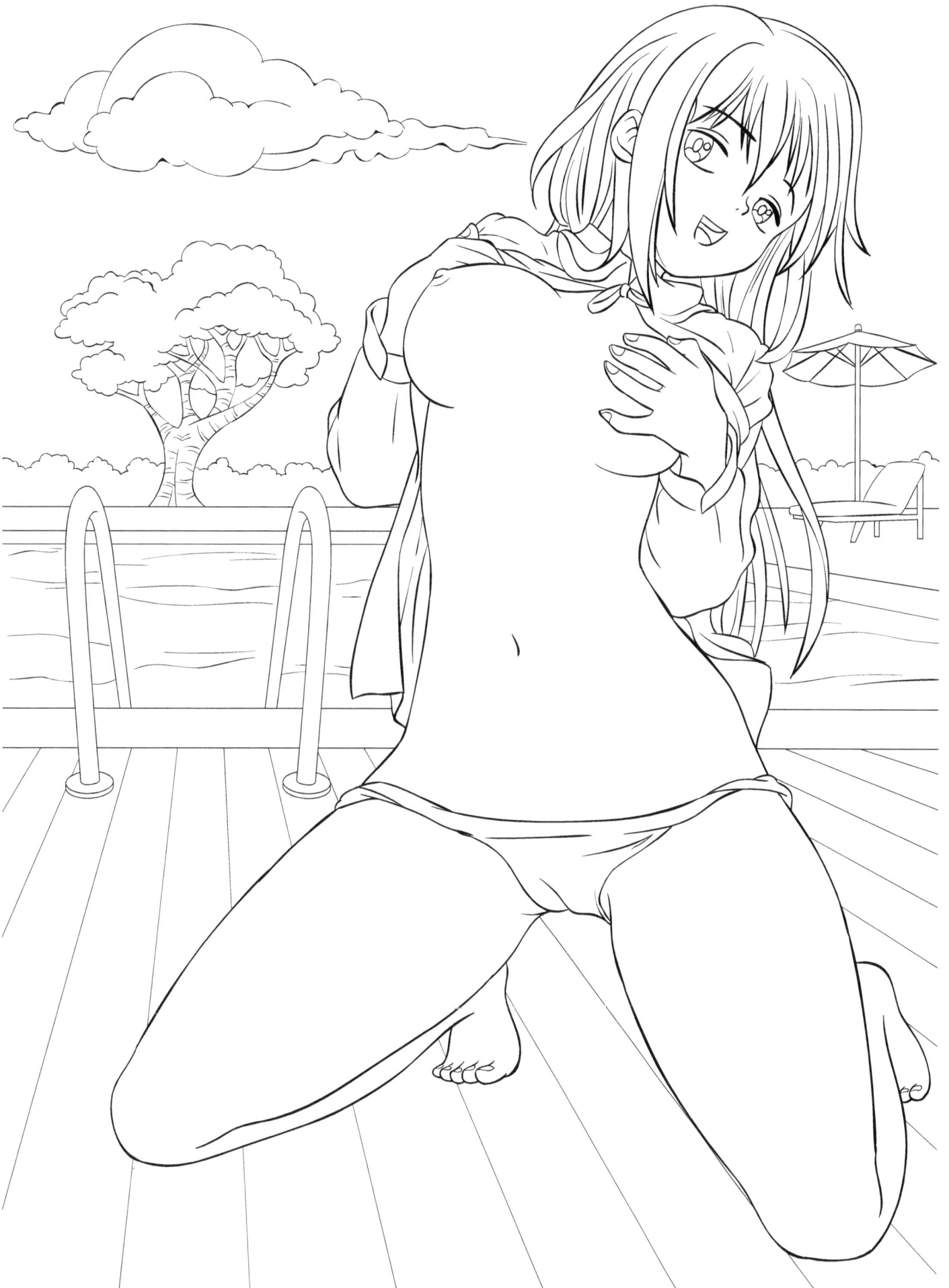

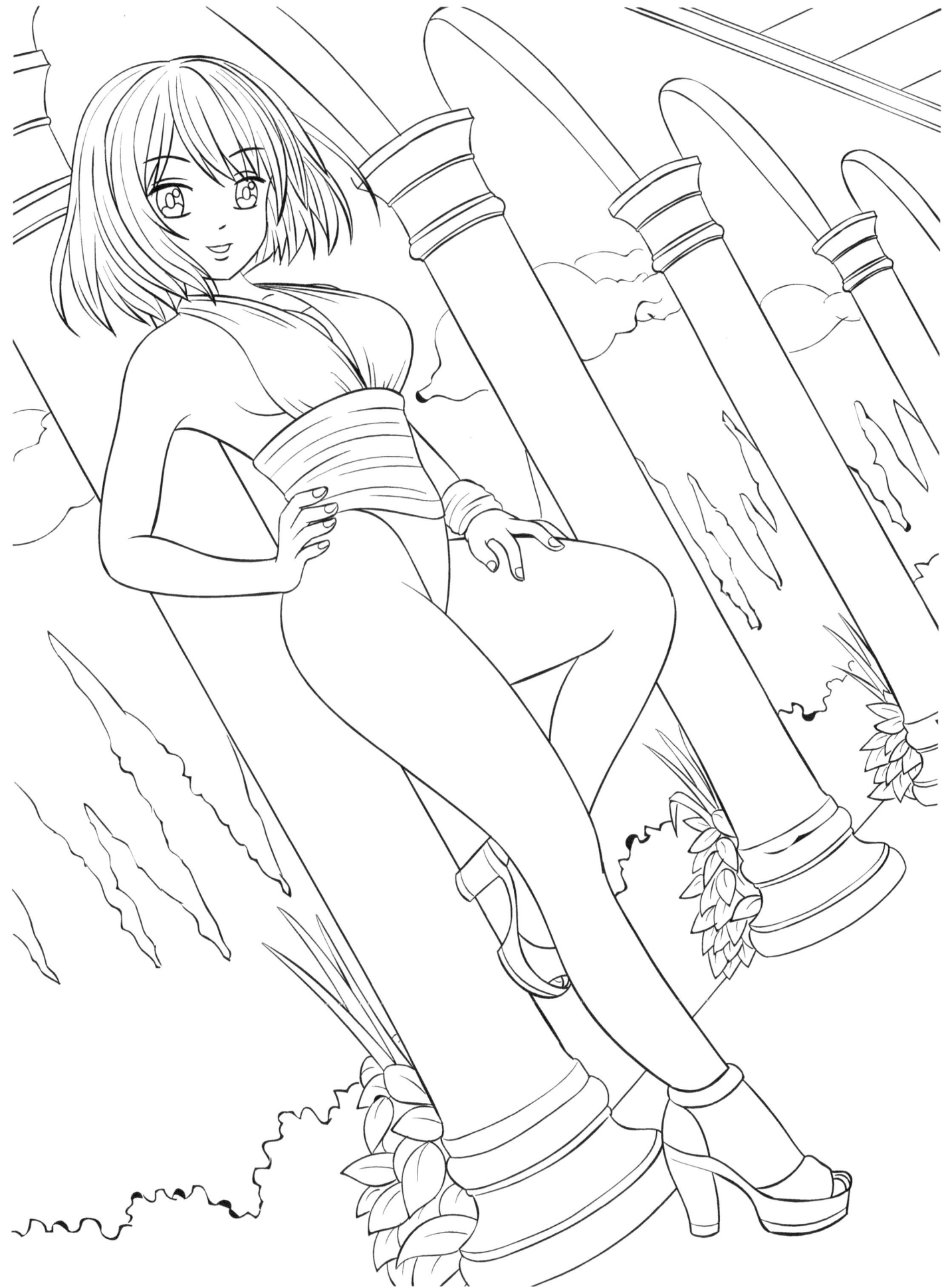

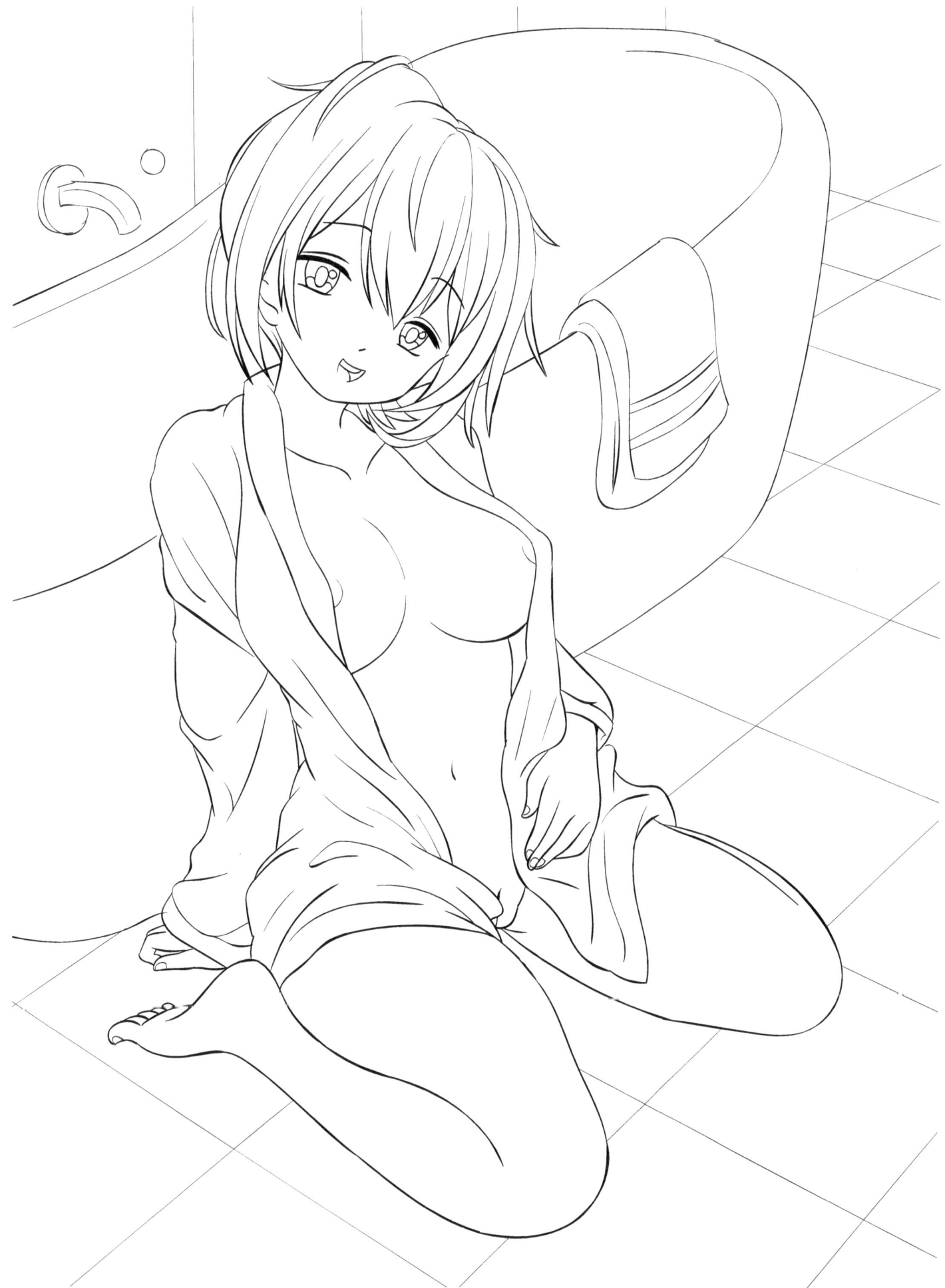

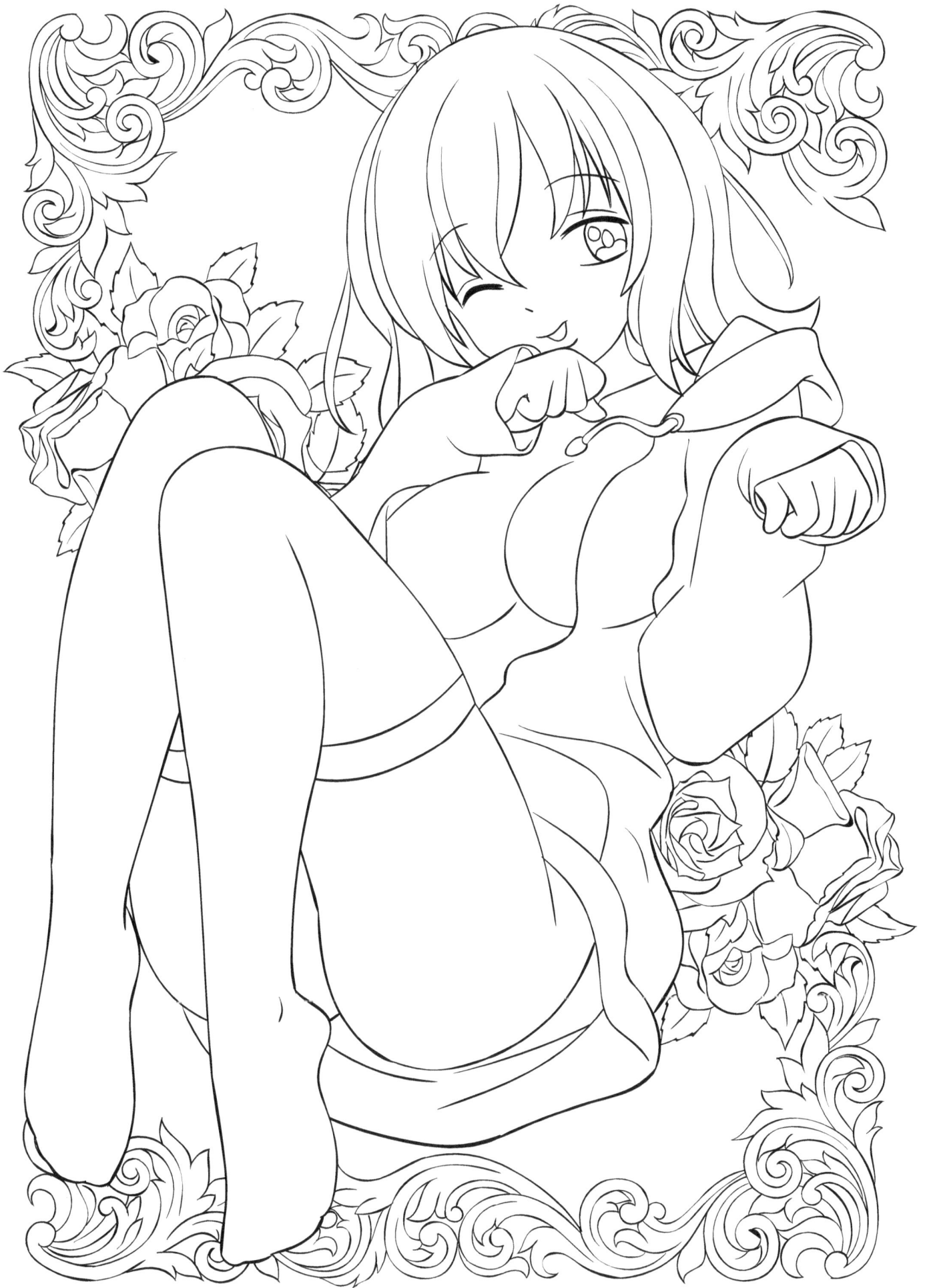

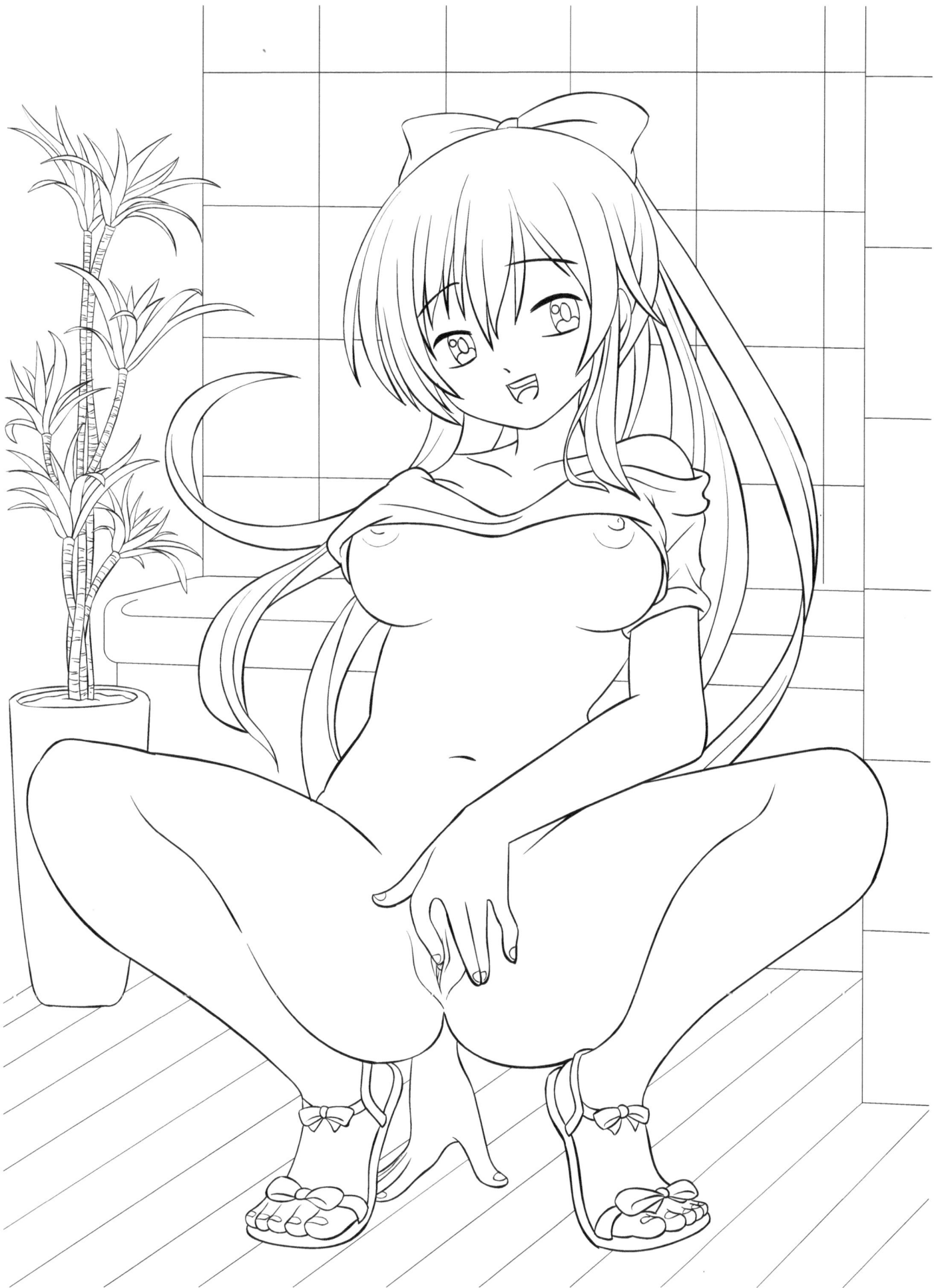

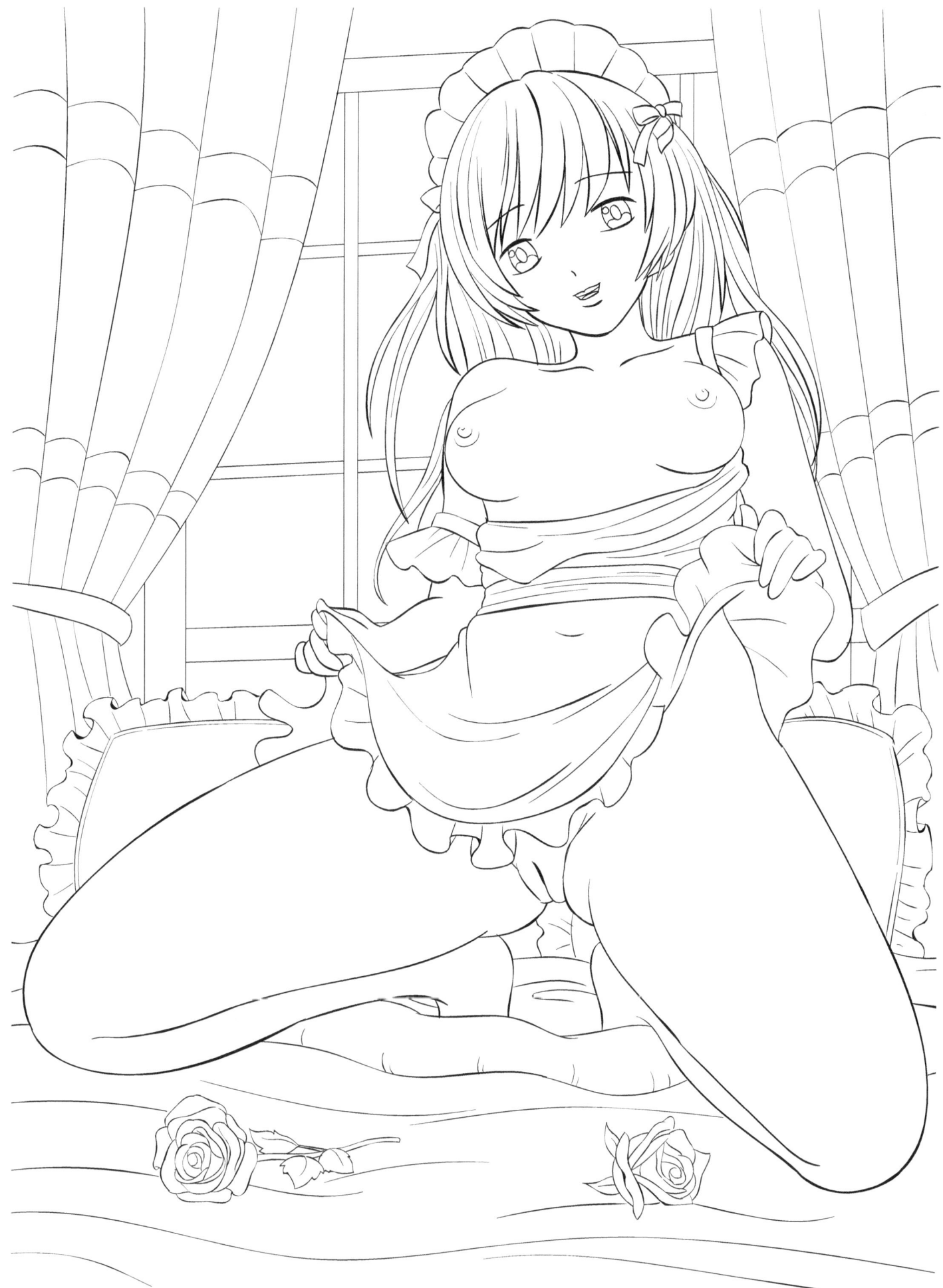

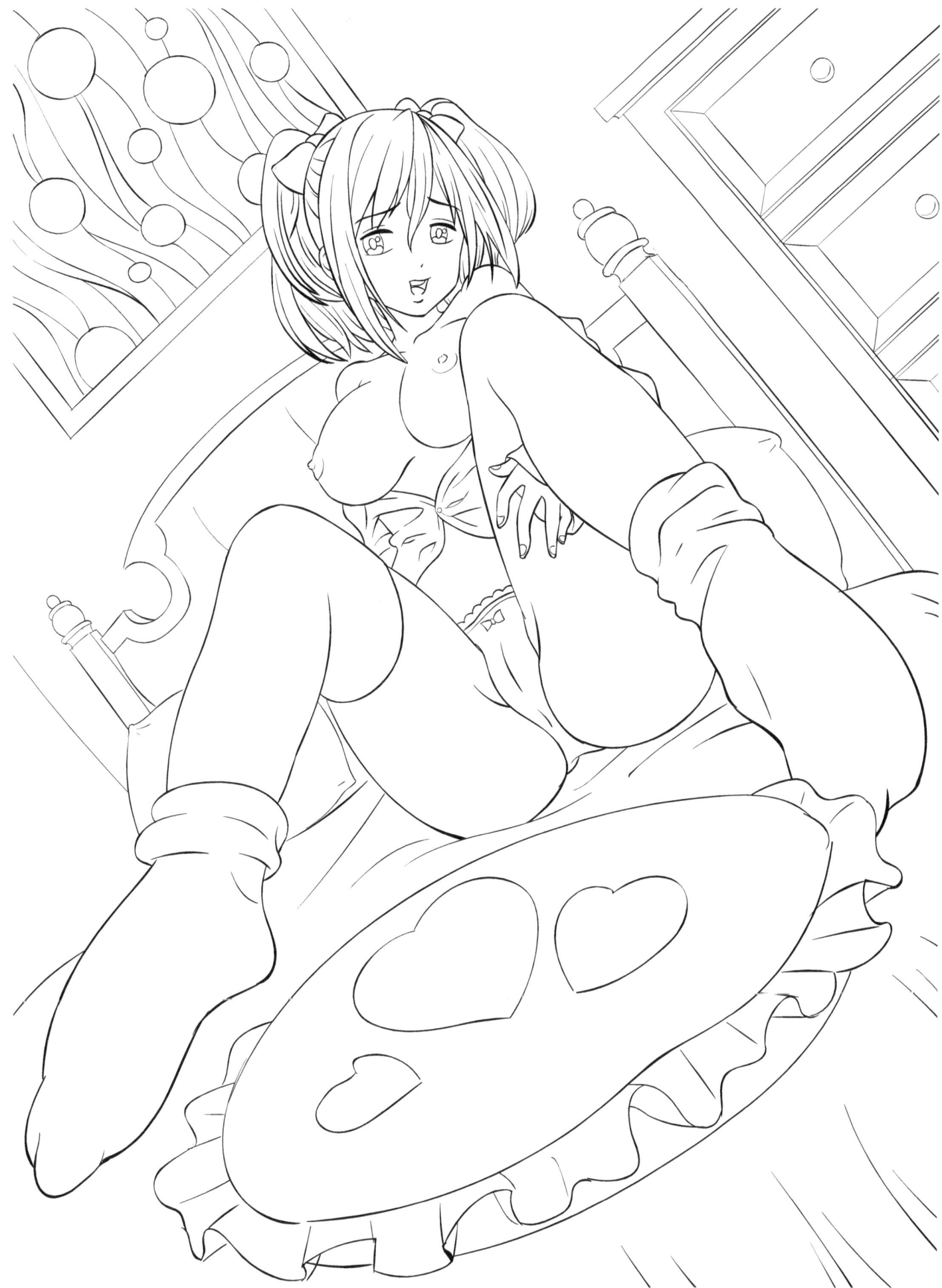

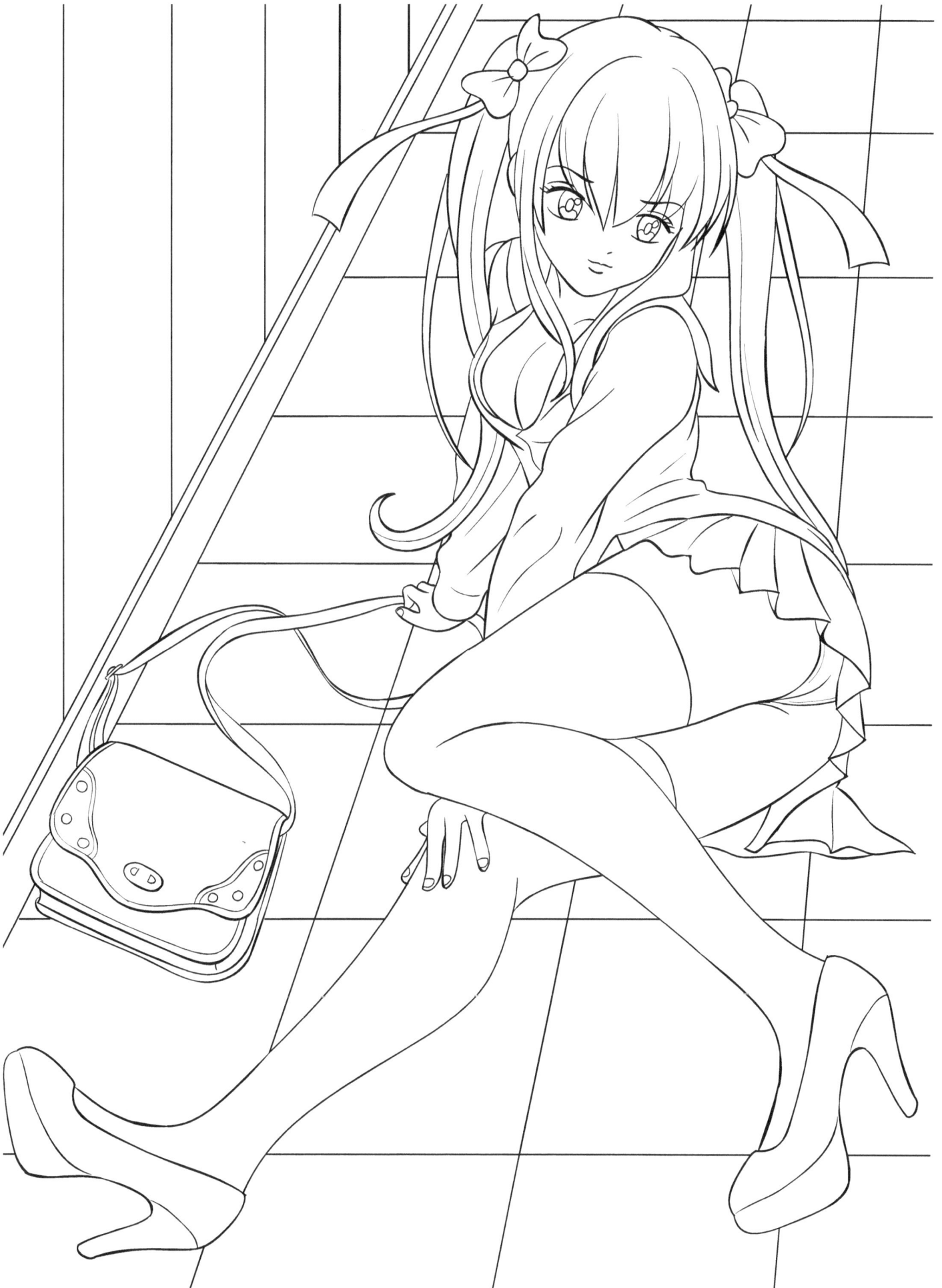

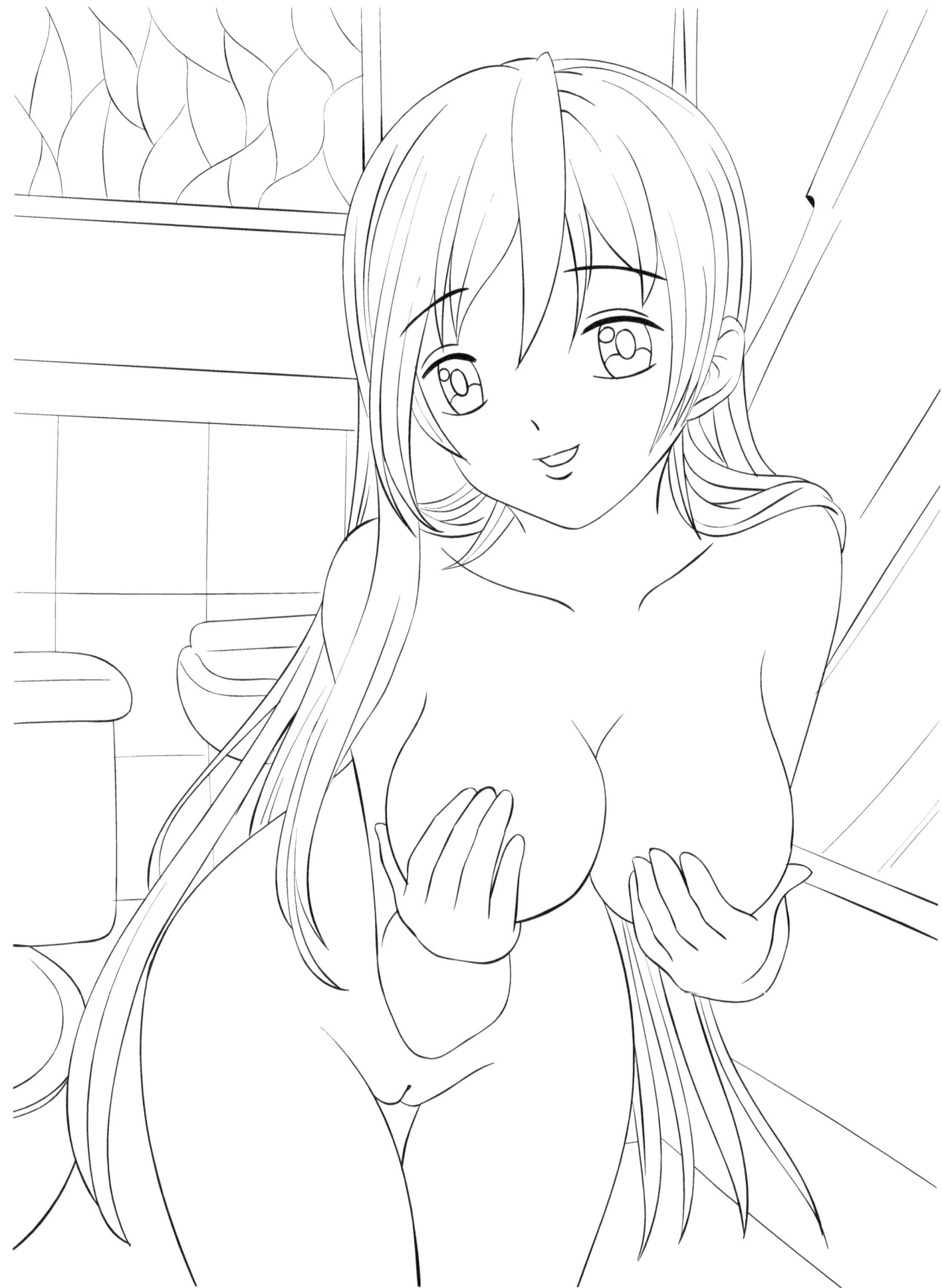

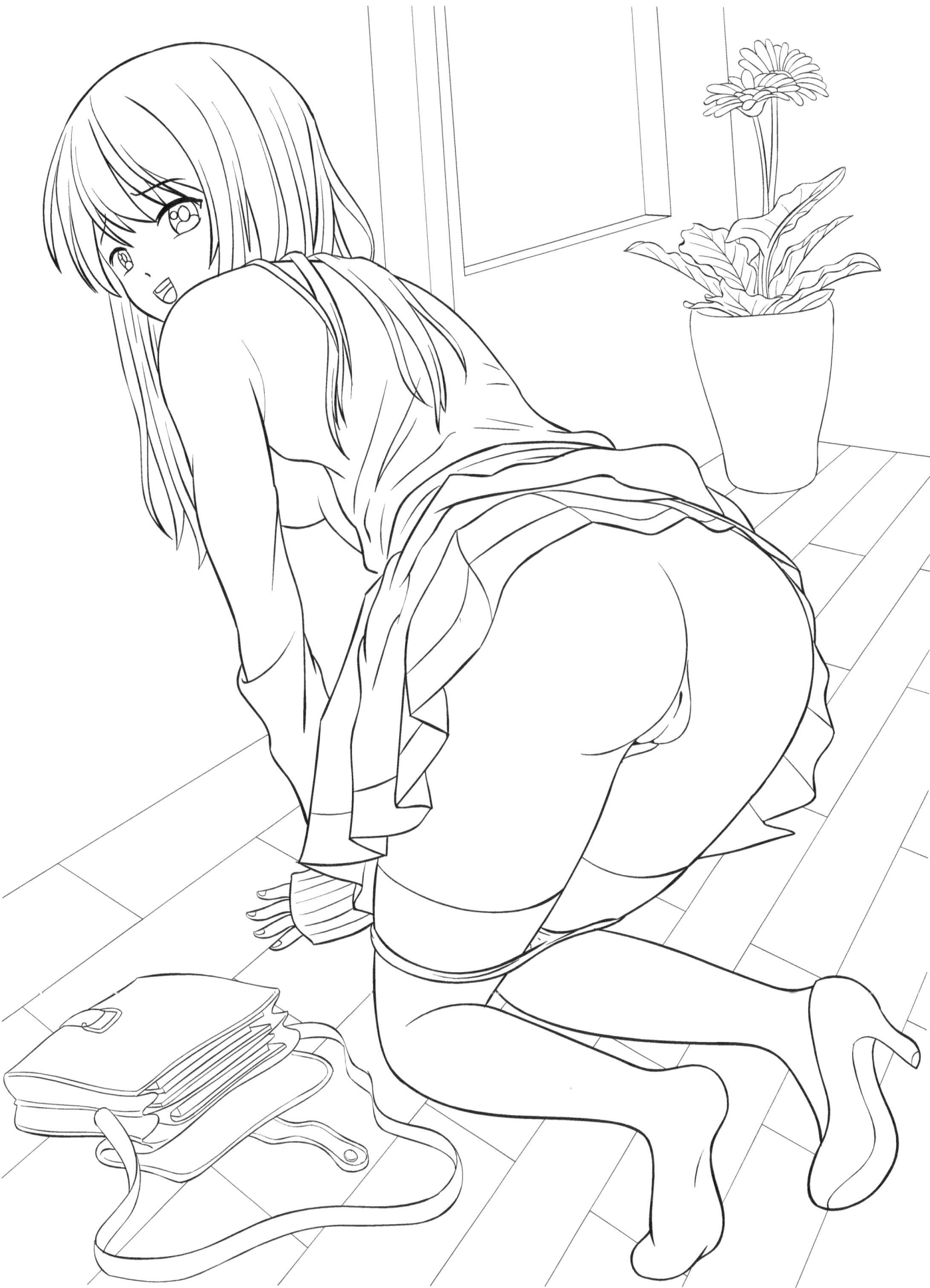

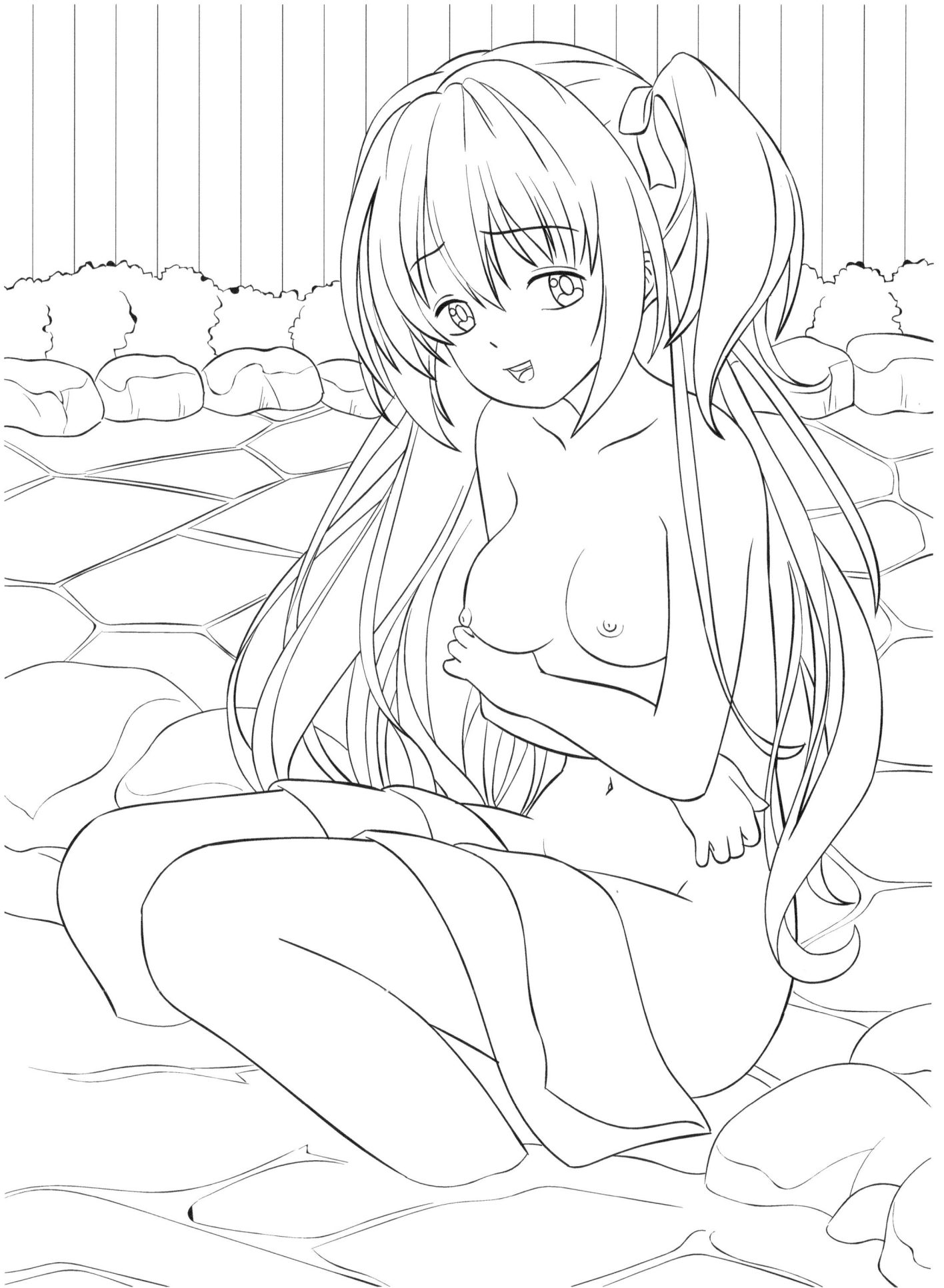

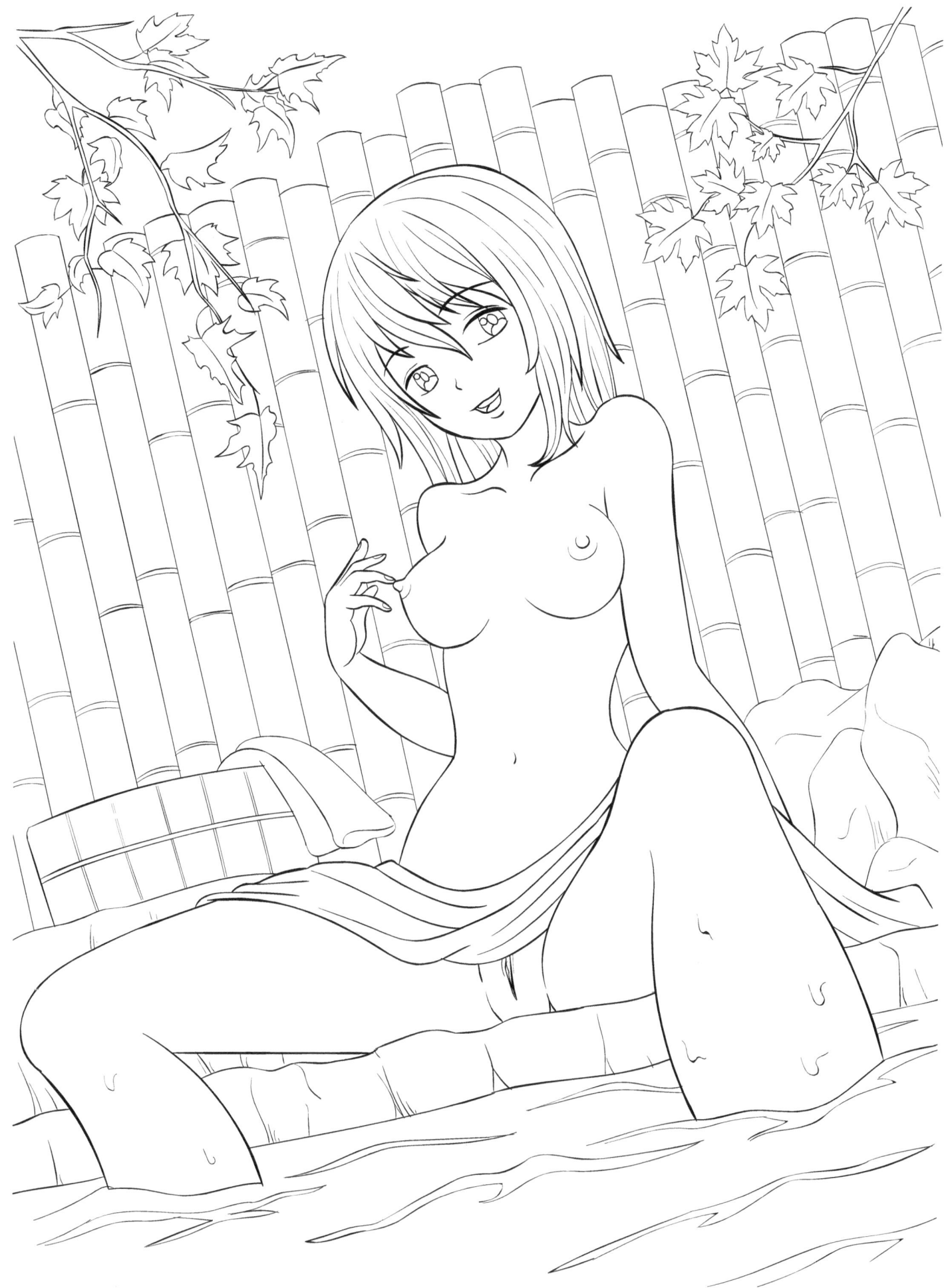

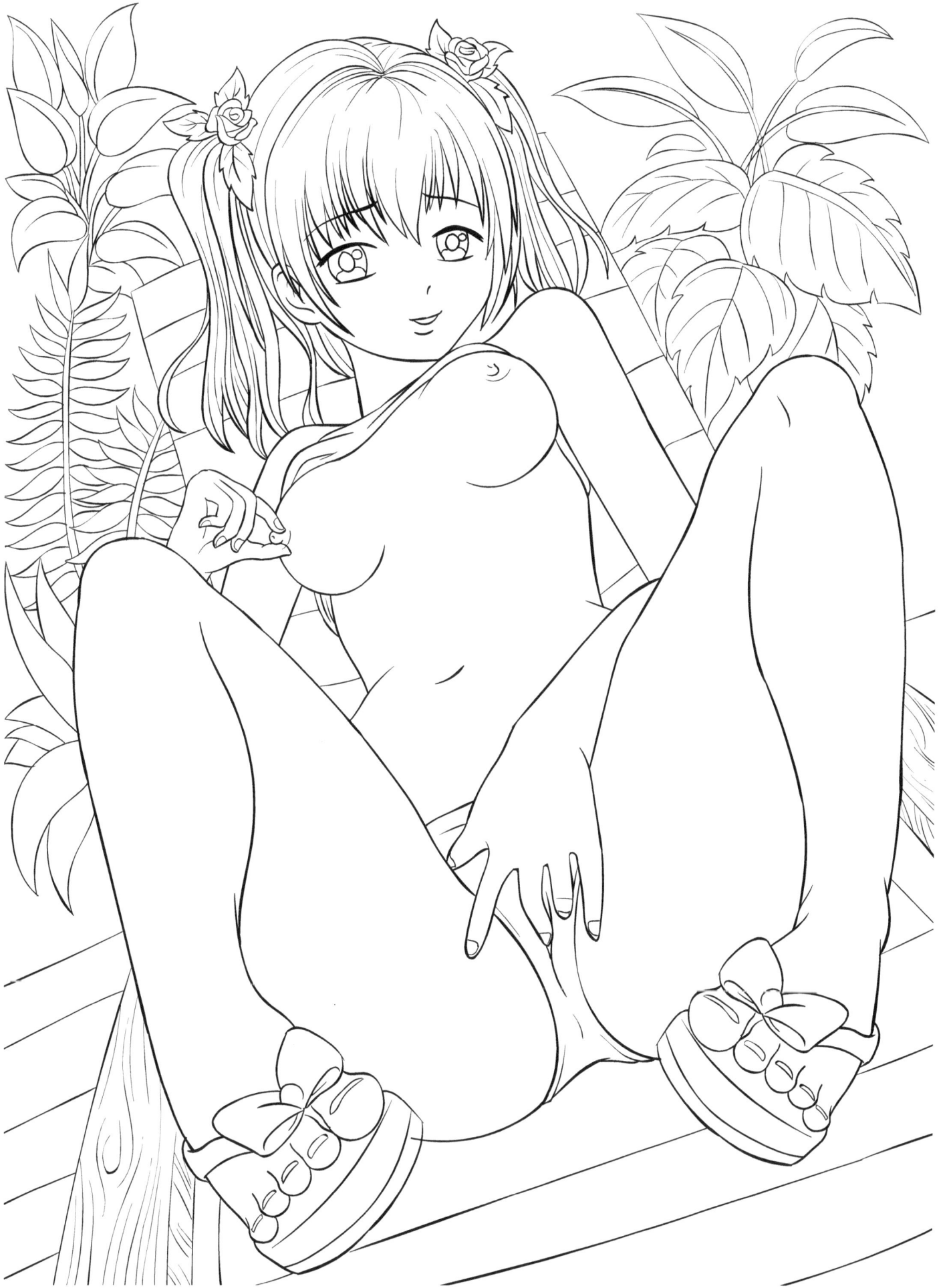

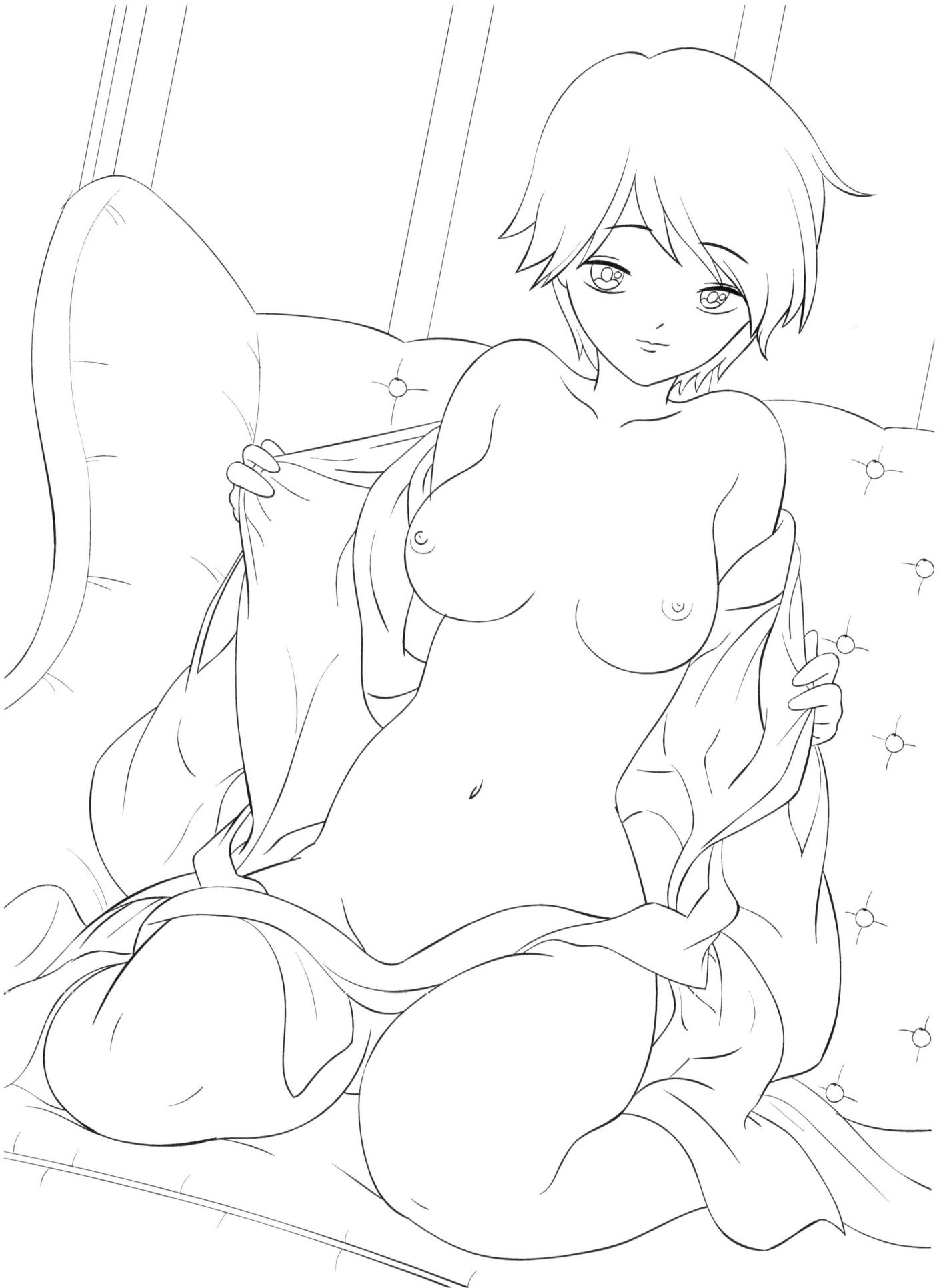

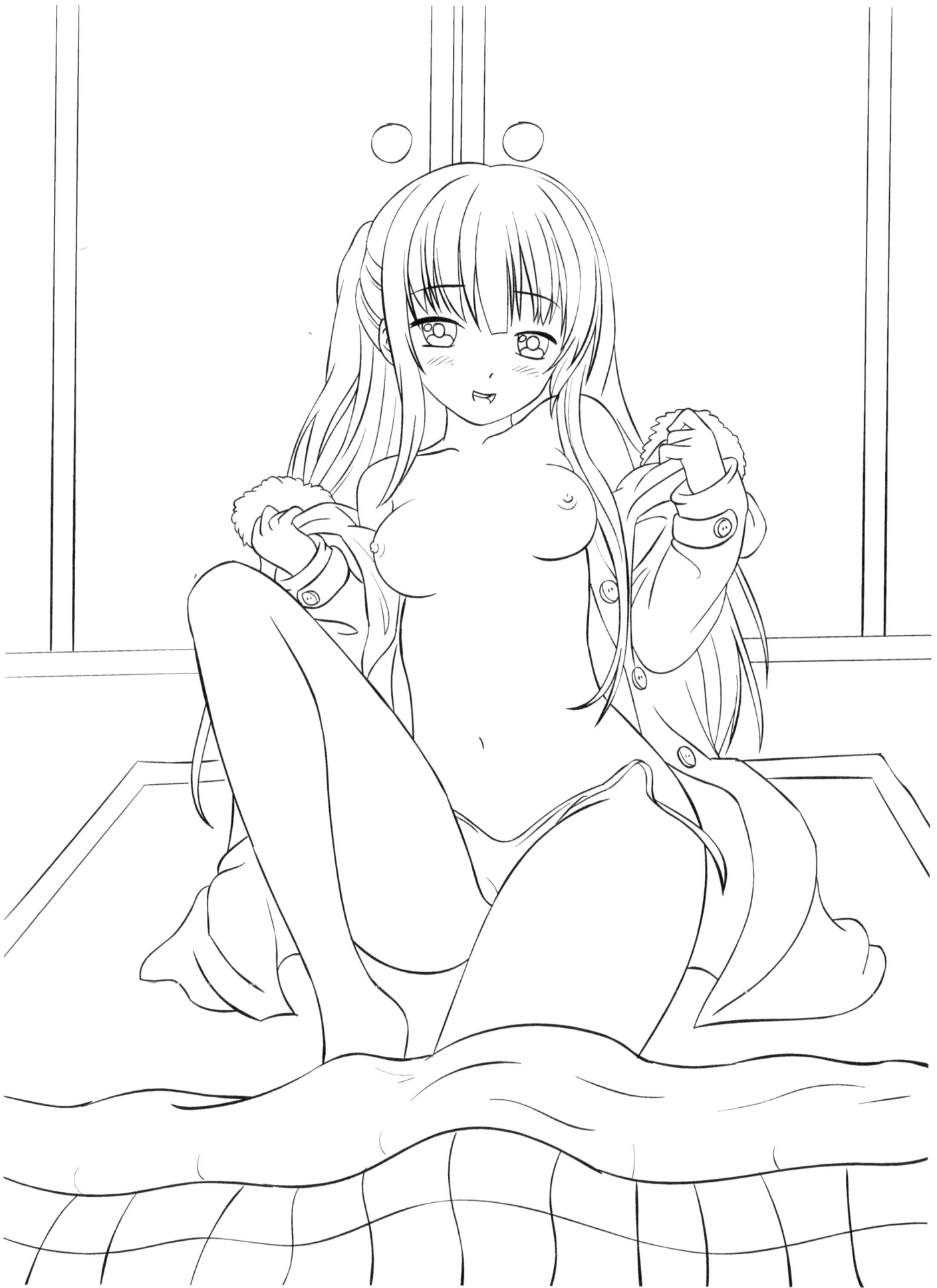

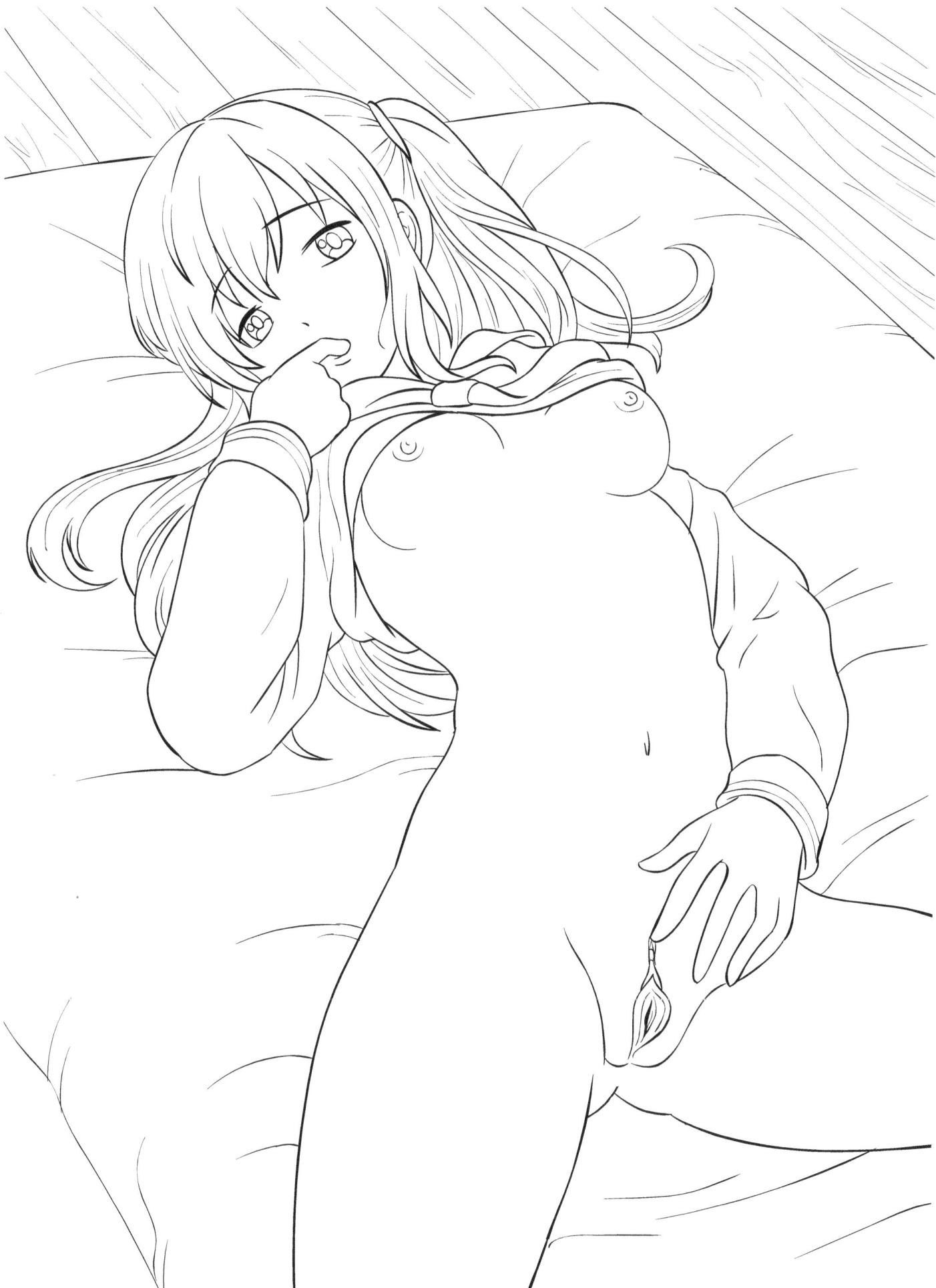

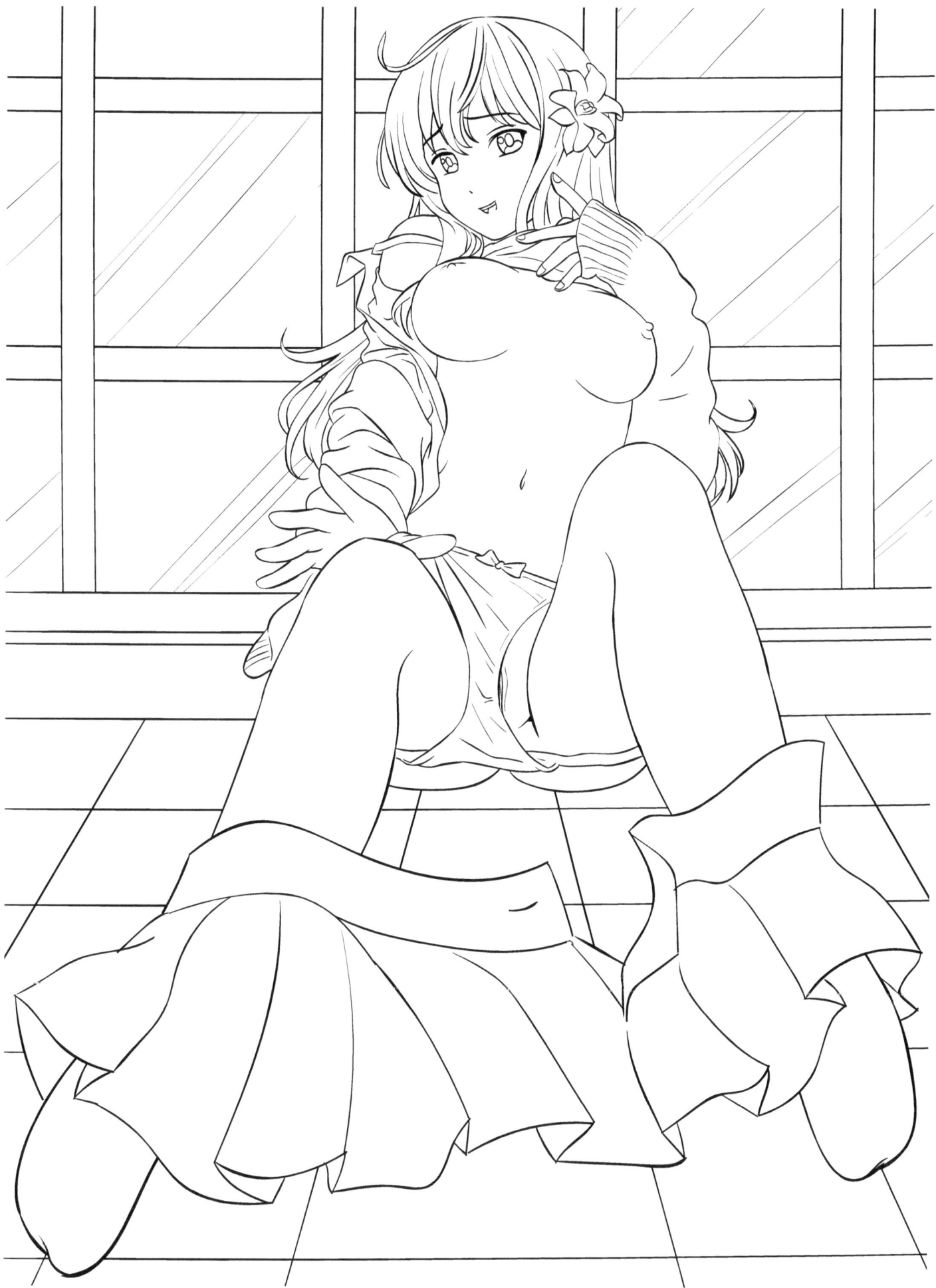

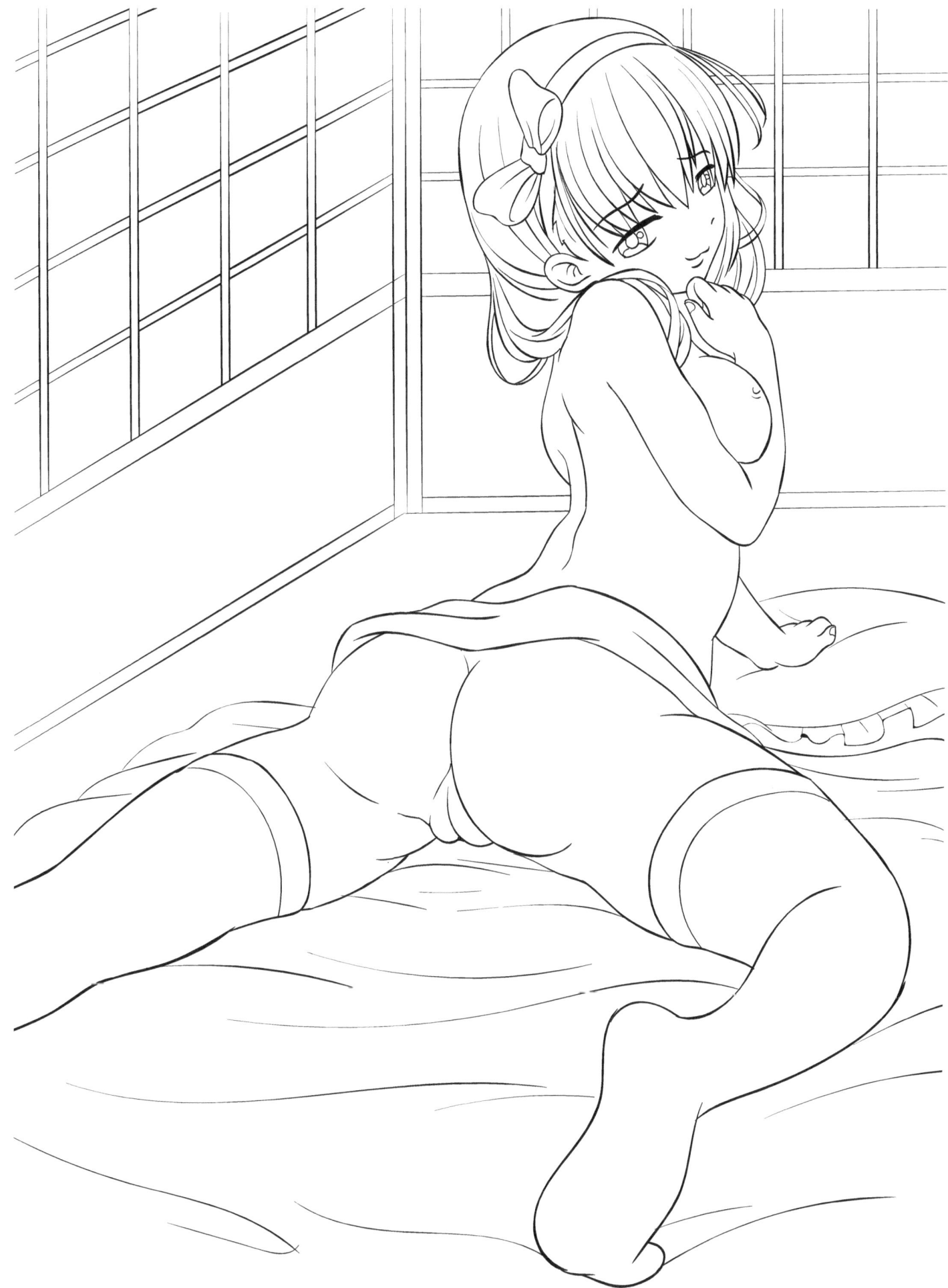

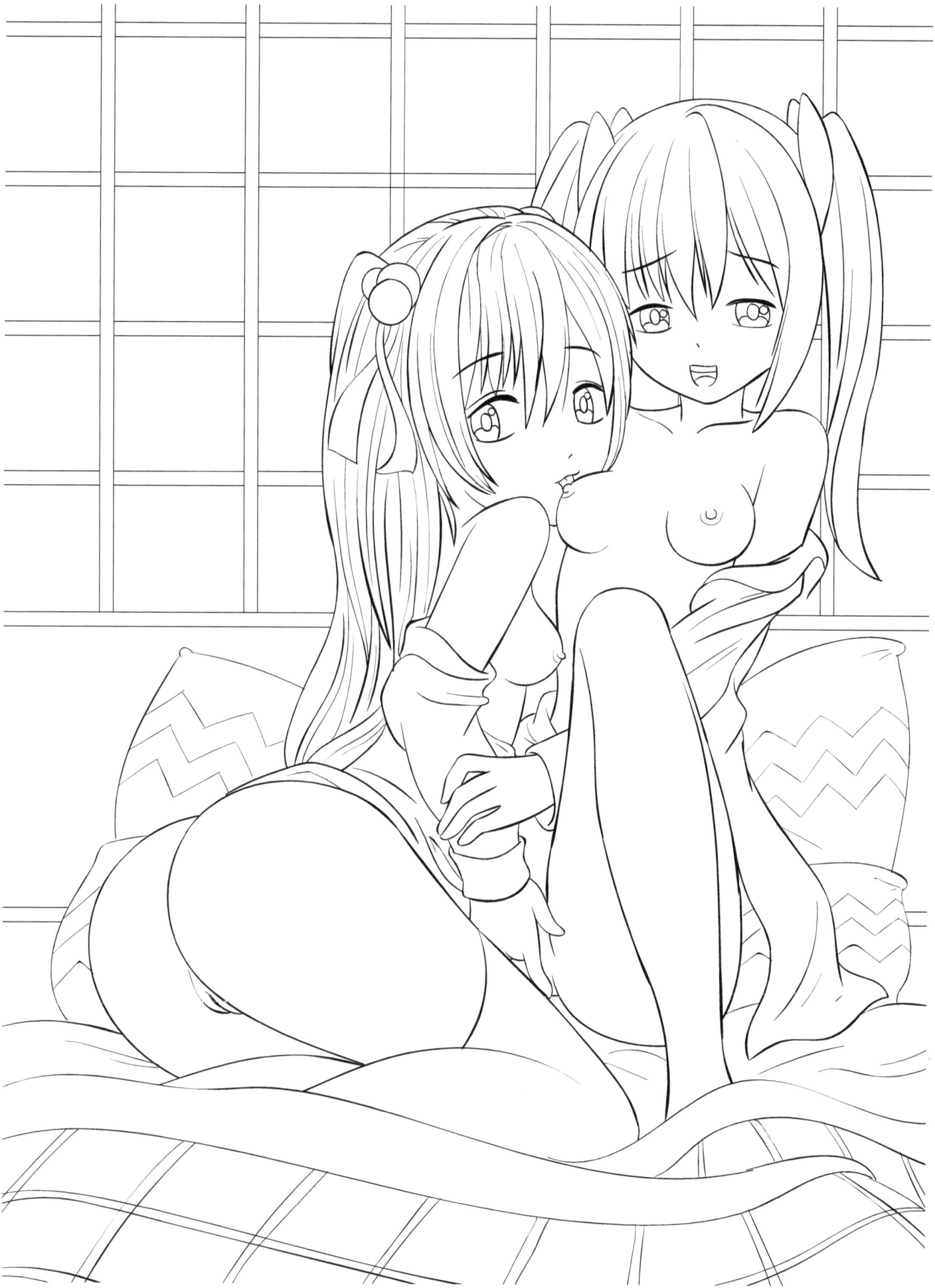

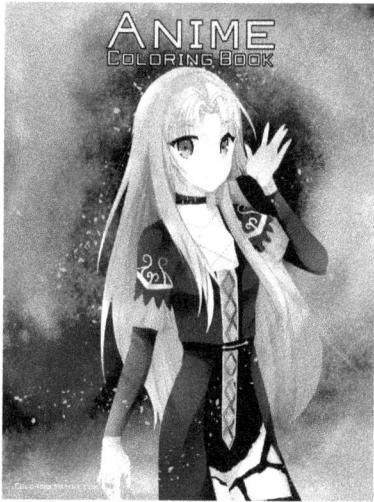
Anime Coloring Book 1

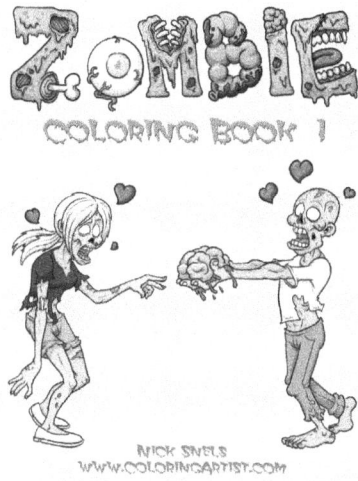
Zombie Coloring Book 1

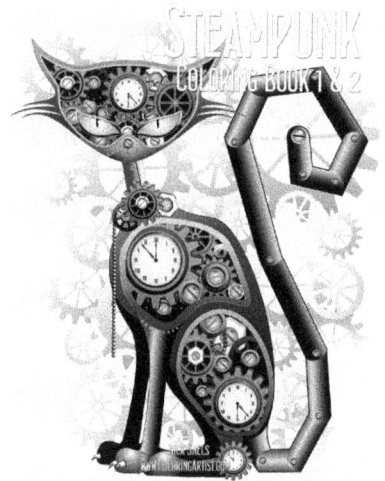
Steampunk Coloring Book 1 & 2

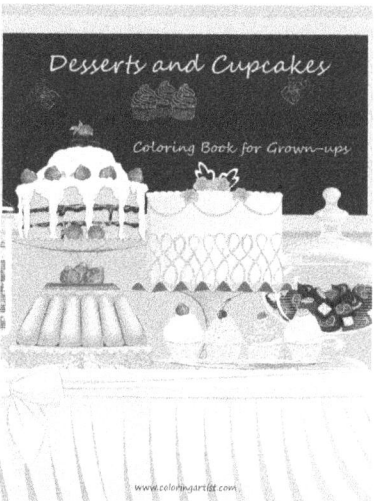
Desserts and Cupcakes
Coloring Book for Grown-Ups 1

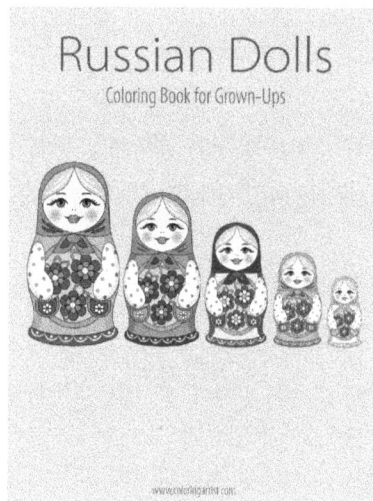
Russian Dolls
Coloring Book for Grown-Ups 1

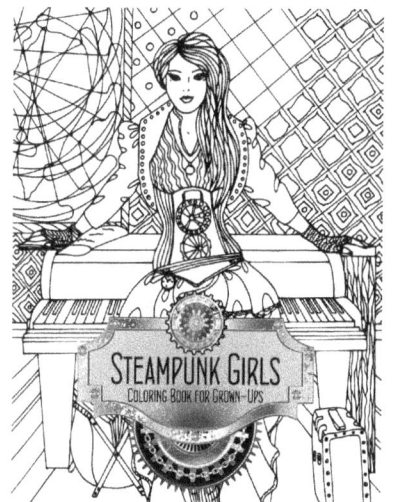
Steampunk Girls
Coloring Book for Grown-Ups 1

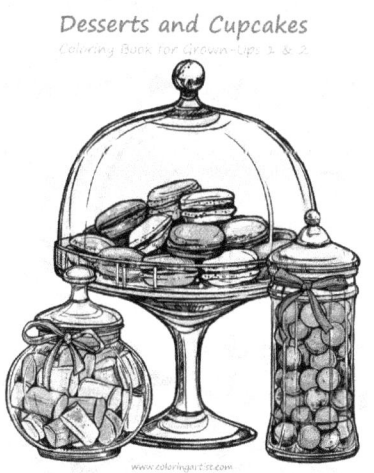
Desserts and Cupcakes
Coloring Book for Grown-Ups 1 & 2

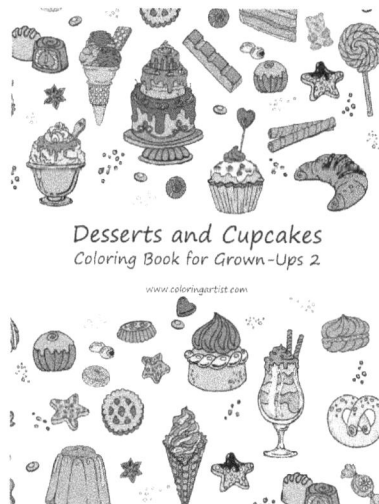
Desserts and Cupcakes
Coloring Book for Grown-Ups 2

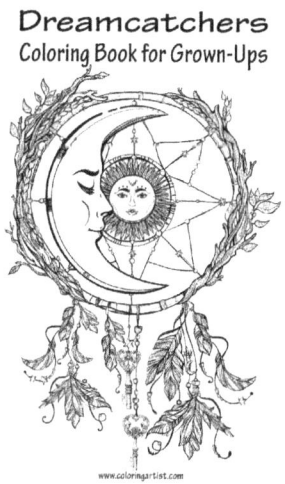
Dreamcatchers
Coloring Book for Grown-Ups 1

Please post a positive review on Amazon,
if you loved this coloring book.

Thank you,

Nick

www.ingramcontent.com/pod-product-compliance
Lightning Source LLC
Chambersburg PA
CBHW051345290326
41933CB00042B/3239